Decoding Your Emotional Appetite

Praise for Molly Zemek

"Taking Molly's course has been the best thing I have done for myself in many years. From the first week, I was able to get rid of my afternoon snacking binges and replace that habit with doing things that take my life in the direction that I want it to go. Also, I was sleeping better, had better digestion, and was happier. This course is everything that I hoped it would be, and much more; it would not be an exaggeration to say that it has been life-changing."
—**Carolyn**, Boothbay, ME

"I lost about forty pounds, so there are inches and clothing sizes that disappeared, but something unanticipated I have noticed is that I don't really hurt anymore when I wake up. Really, my whole mindset about weight and body has changed. I had started several diets and weight loss programs before, but I never really worked on my thoughts around food."
—**Phil**, Roswell, NM

"Eight weeks ago, I started coaching with Molly, and I have lost twenty pounds. My new goal weight is twenty-five pounds (and maybe thirty!). I am feeling fantastic! My energy has increased, my digestive issues have disappeared, and I am really enjoying the process of becoming the future me—the older woman who is healthy, good-looking, and content with herself."
—**Ellen**, Bethesda, MD

"Molly's program was transformative for me. Although I signed up for weight-loss coaching, it was actually the start of a much more important journey to more deeply knowing and appreciating myself. When I started working with Molly, I avoided planning anything in my life more than six months in the future, and I was very resistant to food planning. Molly helped me shift my perspective on planning, transforming it from something oppressive to an act of loving self-care. Growing up, I split my time between the United States and France and learned to really appreciate food. I picked Molly because I wanted to work with someone who loved food as much as I did—without overeating."

—**Amanda**, Claremont, CA

"The physical transformation for me was certainly the weight loss. I also finally (for the first time since I started my diet journey) found a way of eating I can live with. This is a different kind of weight-loss program. Molly takes a holistic approach to changing your relationship with food, as well as changing your approach to life."

—**Yvette**, Oxford, OH

"Working with Molly transformed my thinking around weight loss. I had not dieted much in my life, but I had many preconceived notions, most of which I now realize were not helpful. Molly teaches deep curiosity without judgment, and that is precisely the coaching I needed to reset my life path toward a healthy weight and mindset that will be with me for the rest of my life."

—**Donna**, Carmel, CA

"Working with Molly has been incredible for me. I am down about ten pounds since starting with her, although I consider my mental transformation my biggest achievement. She helped empower me to make huge changes that are effectively changing all aspects of my life. When I felt I had no "me time," she helped to change my mindset and see that I can make changes. When I felt like I "messed up" and fell off the wagon, she treated it as an experiment and a learning opportunity, and I actually do that now! I don't beat myself up when I eat something off plan; I analyze and move on."

—**Lauren**, Hummelstown, PA

"I lost the ten pounds I set out to lose, but my biggest accomplishment is feeling more confident. I have much less anxiety surrounding special events that involve eating because I know I can make choices that serve my body. Investing in yourself is 100 percent worth it. This program is so different from any of the other diet/exercise programs for weight loss I've done since I was fourteen years old. It's been easier to lose ten pounds just by changing my thoughts around food than it has been to count calories, measure food, restrict certain foods, and excessively exercise."

—**Maggie**, Washington, DC

Decoding
Your
EMOTIONAL
APPETITE

A FOOD LOVER'S GUIDE
TO WEIGHT LOSS

MOLLY ZEMEK

NEW YORK

LONDON • NASHVILLE • MELBOURNE • VANCOUVER

Decoding Your Emotional Appetite

A Food Lover's Guide to Weight Loss

Published in New York, New York, by Morgan James Publishing. Morgan James is a trademark of Morgan James, LLC. www.MorganJamesPublishing.com

Proudly distributed by Publishers Group West®

In order to protect client confidentiality, names and identifying details in client stories have been changed

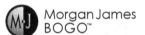

Morgan James BOGO™

A **FREE** ebook edition is available for you or a friend with the purchase of this print book.

CLEARLY SIGN YOUR NAME ABOVE

Instructions to claim your free ebook edition:
1. Visit MorganJamesBOGO.com
2. Sign your name CLEARLY in the space above
3. Complete the form and submit a photo of this entire page
4. You or your friend can download the ebook to your preferred device

ISBN 9781636982601 paperback
ISBN 9781636982618 ebook
Library of Congress Control Number: 2023941605

Cover & Interior Design by:
Christopher Kirk
www.GFSstudio.com

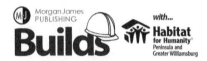

Morgan James PUBLISHING

Builds with... **Habitat for Humanity®** Peninsula and Greater Williamsburg

Morgan James is a proud partner of Habitat for Humanity Peninsula and Greater Williamsburg. Partners in building since 2006.

Get involved today! Visit: www.morgan-james-publishing.com/giving-back

To my family of food lovers: Alex, Peter, Luke, and Andrew.
Thank you for all your love, support, and inspiration.

I cannot count the good people I know who in my mind would be even better if they bent their spirits to the study of their own hungers.

M.F.K. Fisher (1908–1992), food writer

Dear Reader,

I invite you to have a seat beside me at this table to partake in a sensual feast. I will be here, along with your old friend, food, sitting right beside you. We are here for the momentous occasion of celebrating you. Using some of my favorite ingredients, I've cooked up a menu that is so satisfying, it will fill your heart, mind, and soul in a way you've never been nourished before. Course after course, you are welcome to nibble, taste, and savor the layers of flavor in your relationship with food. Delight in the ingredients that resonate with you and leave behind any morsels that are not to your liking. It is all here to enrich your love of yourself and food in a way that serves you best. Nothing is off the table as you dine with us, so pull up your chair, breathe in the scent of your most beloved childhood meal, and prepare your heart for fullness.

xo,

Contents

Introduction:

The Struggle

It seems to me that our three basic needs,
for food and security and love, are so entwined
that we cannot think of one without the other.
M.F.K. Fisher (1908–1992)

Our relationship with food is a lifelong one. From the moment of conception, we depend on our mother for sustenance, and the bond is strengthened when we are held as infants and simultaneously provided milk. The link between safety, comfort, care, and nourishment is deeply rooted in our subconscious from childhood. At an age when we are incapable of feeding ourselves, food becomes love when a caretaker holds us and lifts milk to our mouths. There is warmth, flesh on flesh, and the release of pleasure in our brains when our most primitive needs are met.

1

If you could remember your earliest moments of life, you'd know that something was pulling you toward it from the beginning—a primal hunger to fill a void that only nourishment could satisfy. Before you knew the words for what you needed, the inner language of your emotions spoke for you in reverberations throughout your body. The physical sensation of hunger set off a chain reaction in your being and through crying, fussing, and bringing your tiny fist to your mouth, you sent signals out into the world expressing this desire.

The world responded. Before you could solidify the memory, the connection between food and care was imprinted deep within you. Food became your lifeline, not just for growth and survival, but also for human connection and love. It was always meant to be that way. Through the sound of your mother's voice, the warmth of her body against yours, the unique scent of her close by, the smooth and milky sweetness of your earliest food, eating was a sensorial experience creating pleasure.

Within the first year of life, like all babies, you started absorbing the world around you. Through your eyes, you made connections about what people do, how they express themselves, and where food fits into the equation. With your ears, you made sense of sounds and words, and with your hands, you put everything together in your mouth to understand the shape and taste of life around you. You grew, and with maturity, you noticed that food is not simply what's consumed for nourishment or a means to satisfy hunger. It is how we connect with one another around a table, how we have fun in front of the TV, or how we quell boredom. Maybe as a child you learned that fussiness is quieted with a bag of Cheerios, and in kindergarten, graham crackers and apple juice were a midday ritual that comforted you before naptime.

Take a moment now and reflect on your earliest recollection of food and the rituals of eating it for comfort. How old were you? Who provided food and what role did it serve? Perhaps you remember a particular routine that involved eating outside of a regular mealtime. Consider the feelings that come up when you reflect on that memory. It's possible your brain made a connection between eating and feeling comforted and safe. Maybe you had an experience where there was not enough food to go around, and you feel a sense of lack or urgency when you recall those early memories of eating. These emotional imprints likely stayed with you as you grew and matured. They may now form the backbone of your current relationship with food.

Relationship expert and author Gary Chapman popularized the concept of love languages with his book *The Five Love Languages: The Secret to Love That Lasts*. I would like to add one more: The love language of food begins before we have the words to speak our desire for it. It is a heartfelt connection, so primal and multifaceted that to deny it would be to reject the essence of life itself.

Eating is one way we express and experience love for ourselves and care for our bodies. But in society, it's also a way that we connect and share our love with others. Understanding this at a basic level makes it easy to see how easily food can become something we depend on for reasons other than physical nourishment—how it can soothe emotional pain, fill the void of loneliness, and pretend to take care of us in the absence of natural self-care. Like any relationship that becomes toxic, an overreliance on food beyond what is helpful, healthful, or heartfelt erodes our relationship with it and compromises our relationship with ourselves in the process.

You might have picked up this book because these days you feel like you have no control around food. The tug-of-war in your mind between what you want to eat and what you should eat is so exhausting that it's easier to surrender to another bowl of ice cream at the end of the day. It's understandable that you feel frustrated when you believe it's your fault or should just have more self-control.

The truth is that nothing is wrong with you. Your relationship with food is a complex one that developed before you had the awareness to understand it. Maybe it was obligatory snack breaks on the soccer field during your elementary years, regular trips to McDonald's, or traditional holiday meals abundant with all the possibilities. Whatever your unique memories are, food seemed to just appear, and the choice was easy.

To understand why food no longer feels like an easy choice for you, we can begin by gently tugging at one thread and tracing your history with food until we untangle it, like a ball of yarn. What seems like a simple decision to lift a bite of food to your mouth begins first with a thought. The thoughts you formulate in your mind are always the source of the choices you make in your relationship with food.

The power lies with you.

For years, I believed that food had the upper hand. That my struggle with overeating was not the result of my thinking but the result of food itself. I believed that food was too irresistible, too tempting. There are countless dieting regimes that further convinced me of this truth. I just needed to eat the right foods, in the right quantities, and eliminate the rest. Or maybe I just needed to eat more often, in smaller amounts, and never experience hunger. I used to believe that the solution lay in following one of these prescribed plans and getting the weight off. But I always intended to go back to my old friend, food. Dieting was a means to be able to overeat again without sacrificing my figure in the process. This began the dance of deprivation, and in turn the overindulgence that followed.

Looking outside myself for the solution to overeating always made food the culprit. To be clear, there are no guilty parties here. There is me, and there is you, dear reader. We are the ones who learned ways to relate to food from a young age. We are the ones who unknowingly adapted to the messaging of society and consumed things without understanding why or being aware of the habits created in the process.

Life happened, food appeared, we responded.

Of course, it is more complicated than that, and the aim of this book is to help you understand the unique patterns formed in your relationship with food. These patterns form your emotional appetite, and learning to decode that appetite will put you back in touch with your body. Learning to listen to the language of your body and its true physical appetite is how you address the core of what you need to feel well beyond food.

It's important to note that there are still many impoverished people in this world who lack basic food and nutrition. A portion of the proceeds from this book will go directly to the global charity *Feed the Hungry*. I also want to mention that this book does not intend to address those diagnosed with eating disorders.

While my hope is that these stories help you cultivate mindfulness around eating, they don't take the place of advice from a medical professional.

What I've learned is that food is not a guilty party. Food just sits there. It didn't ask to go into your mouth. It didn't force its way in. It didn't call your name. Food has no moral value until we decide it does. It's not good, bad, right, or wrong, and labeling it is problematic. When food is "good" or "bad," what does it say about the person consuming it?

Placing blame on food or yourself is messy, and it doesn't help the process of unraveling the patterns you created over time. Understanding yourself and rediscovering your power over food involves accepting that nothing has gone wrong. If you struggle with eating more than you want, or not eating enough, let's begin with accepting where you are. I can meet you on the road you're traveling and help you retrace the steps that brought you here. In the end, these steps will lead you back to yourself.

I often tell prospective clients who come to me for help with weight loss that their external goal of shedding pounds is inevitable if they use the tools I provide. But what they don't realize is that their outer transformation is often less rewarding than what changes on the inside. The real prize they create for themselves is a stronger relationship with self. When I told one of my clients, Sherry, this, she immediately blew it off.

"Yeah, yeah, that's fine," she said, "but I'm really only interested in getting to my goal weight." Like most people, Sherry believed that food was the problem, and that weight loss was the solution. Three months after completing my course, she was amazed by her newfound confidence. Not only had she lost twenty pounds, but she no longer thought about food or her body in the same way.

"My life is about so much more than food now," she said on a call with me. "I'm enjoying myself in a way I never have before."

Over the course of the next several chapters, I will invite you into the lives of Sherry and many other clients who explored their relationship with food with me during my coaching program *Weight Loss for Food Lovers*. I created the program after discovering the solution to my own battle with overeating and realizing that food was never the problem.

My journey involved recounting my own love affair with food, from growing up in a family of food lovers to a career as a professional chef, and how I lost myself along the way. I was my first client, and when I finally lost forty-five pounds in a way that seemed easy and natural, it felt like true freedom. I knew I needed to share the process with other food lovers who felt stuck in a relationship they did not fully comprehend. I decided to get certified as a life and weight loss coach so I could guide others through the same path of self-discovery. It was the beginning of my business Molly Zemek Coaching and my signature program *Weight Loss for Food Lovers*.

My story is at the heart of this book, because I live the exact process I teach my clients. I have intimate knowledge of the struggle that food lovers face, but I also learned how to navigate my way out. I used my own success to build the foundation of my program, then refined it by hearing the stories of countless others and helping them achieve their own freedom around food.

What emerged were common patterns that form what I call our *emotional appetite*. This appetite includes a spectrum of reasons we turn to food beyond physical hunger. When you can identify your emotional appetite(s) and explore the reasons they formed, you can begin to create more of the relationship you truly want with food and your body. Instead of feeling troubled and confused, you can have the balance you want of nourishing your body, enjoying pleasure, and supporting yourself with love. By decoding your emotional appetite, you can relearn your physical appetite and identify the true desires of your heart. I will help you find your way back to loving yourself. All roads lead to you.

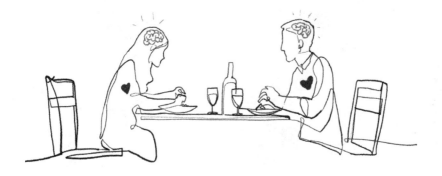

Part I:

The Foundation of
Your Relationship with Food

Chapter 1:

My Story

My earliest memory of food was my first birthday. I am sitting in a wooden highchair wearing a white-smocked dress embroidered with baby chicks. On the tray in front of me sits my very own five-inch birthday cake. It came from the best bakery in town, iced in white buttercream. Around the top are perfectly piped pale-pink roses with leaves peeking out underneath.

I have two pictures of this occasion on my desk, and I am looking at them now as I write this. In the first photo, I stare intently at the confection before me. I must know it's special. It has all my favorite colors, and the flowers, swirls, and candles are all for me. There is no knife or fork close by. This is not for sharing. It is my birthday, and someone must care about me.

In the next picture, I look directly at the camera. My cheeks are smeared with frosting, and crumbs dot my mouth and hands.

There are no other signs of the cake. The tray in front of me is completely clear.

It does not take much to sleuth out what happened. I devoured every bite of my first birthday treat. I used my eyes, my hands, my mouth, and my brain to learn that food was important. It was beautiful, it tasted good, it felt good, and it showed love. It was the beginning of my love affair with food.

My father has Italian heritage, so I understood that food was a love language early on. Over breakfast, he asked, "What's for dinner?" My mother spent several hours each day procuring groceries from a variety of different stores. The meals she cooked were not fancy, but they required the best quality ingredients. Red wine vinegar with 7 percent acidity, seeded multigrain bread, Parmigiano Reggiano stamped in black-dotted print along the rind to show its authenticity, San Marzano crushed tomatoes. Food was something we made time for.

The kitchen, like most homes, was the heart. My mother chopped, diced, and fried. I watched pools of emerald olive oil spill into a pan and shimmer in the heat. Roasted garlic and sautéed onions wafted in the air, and my mother passed me small pieces of meat to nibble as I watched, mesmerized. I was like an obedient puppy, staring expectantly by her side.

When we sat down to eat, it was with the same anticipation. My father's favorite was spaghetti with meat sauce, Granny's salad, and a generous pour of Chianti Classico. When I set the table, I made sure there were always two things: black pepper and crushed red pepper. My father seasoned almost everything with it.

Eating was not simply a mundane necessity, a way to fuel the body for survival. It was always a full-blown sensory experience. In my childhood home, eating was not just what kept us alive. We lived for it.

At dinner, we gave full attention to the food. Around the table of my childhood home in Virginia, sitting down for supper was the moment we anticipated. Curls of steam rose from bowls piled high with a tangle of noodles. A rainbow of celery, carrots, tomatoes, and lettuce filled a wooden salad bowl, and a basket brimmed with ovals of toasted bread slathered in garlicky butter. Years later, when I was enrolled in culinary school, I relearned that "first we eat with our eyes."

Second, we eat with our noses. As I sat with my steaming bowl of spaghetti, the smell of slow-cooked tomatoes rose and hovered around the table. I breathed it in greedily, knowing what was to come. Across the table, my father often tipped his nose in the bulb of a wine glass for one long, drawn-out moment, eyes closed as if in prayer. I was too young to know he was inhaling the history of a faraway country—a country where his relatives pressed wine in their basement and hand-cut gnocchi at the kitchen counter.

Any natural food lover understands that taste and feel work collectively to create the experience your mouth has once that first bite enters. My mother's version of pasta with meat sauce was the recipe she learned watching my father's grandmother, but every meal was an opportunity for critique—a chance to reevaluate and fine-tune. I was ready to taste after spooling a forkful of noodles into a neat spiral covered in sauce.

As a child, I learned to determine the worthiness of each mouthful from my father. The first few bites of every meal, he was silent, considering the flavor and texture in his mouth. Was the pasta al dente, so the spaghetti still had a slight firmness to it? Were the noodles adequately salted and hot enough? I knew the food I ate tasted good, and as a young girl, I learned that sometimes it could even be better with the right ingredients.

My memories of food as a child reveal a relationship with food for pleasure and connection. I equated eating with feeling love from my family. With every bite I put into my small mouth, I assumed feeling good must mean I was loving on myself. There was no reason to stop.

When my father turned forty, he was diagnosed with heart disease, and there was a dramatic shift in our food culture at home. My paternal grandfather died of a heart attack at fifty, so my dad was particularly sensitive to the threat this diagnosis carried. It seemed like overnight he replaced all his favorite foods with fat-free alternatives. He eliminated red meat, fried foods, and most desserts. Within no time, he lost about twenty pounds.

The dialogue in our house expanded to include a new vocabulary. We all became versed in the ten most essential superfoods. Instead of Parmigiano Reggiano, my mom started sourcing out goji berries.

There was new scrutiny toward what we all ate, and ingredients were no longer prioritized for pleasure, but rather for their virtue. Gone were the oversized chocolate chip cookies my father enjoyed for dessert. They were no longer on the "good" list.

This new philosophy was well-intentioned but challenging to swallow. I quickly became self-conscious after growing up immersed in our family's food culture and reveling in the sheer pleasure of taste. It didn't help that I was entering puberty and naturally more aware of body image. I was aware of my mother's desire to count calories and my father's drive toward optimal health, yet I wrestled with my internal passion for food. I had never learned how to eat in moderation and was confused about how to adopt a virtuous relationship with food.

Guilt set in. If food was either good or bad, I deduced that my food choices must somehow reflect my moral character. I felt ashamed to eat "unhealthy" food in front of my parents. I still wanted to clear my plate and follow dinner with dessert, so I started hiding. Not all the time. But when I wanted more, I snuck back into the kitchen and swiped a few more bites while no one was looking. I grabbed another cookie and walked into a different room where no one could see me eat it. I looked for ways to rendezvous with food. It was my guilty pleasure, and an escape.

My parents guided me down a traditional academic path, and I was fortunate enough to attend a college that encouraged me to think for myself. I had a secret dream to abandon my parents' well-intentioned plans and attend culinary school. The idea of sitting at a desk making money could never compete with the thrill of being in a kitchen experimenting with recipes. But as much as my father loved food, he believed cooking was merely a hobby. In his eyes, I had far greater potential.

For fear of disappointing him, I obediently followed the more acceptable path and attended graduate school for Spanish. But instead of studying my coursework, I thumbed through cookbooks and scheduled trips to farmer's markets. I invited fellow graduate students over for three-course meals paired with wine and made notes of how to improve my favorite recipes. But no matter how much I cooked or ate, I couldn't escape the agony of pursuing a career I did not love.

The flame of desire to work as a full-time cook grew slowly on the back burner of my mind until I could no longer deny it. I was miserable, and the only thing that delighted me was cooking. When I should have been analyzing Spanish literature and grading freshman exams, I was working my way through *The Joy of Cooking* and comparing varieties of heirloom tomatoes. I didn't understand how the pleasure of eating helped me escape the depression I felt. I just knew the one part of my life where I experienced passion was with food.

My parents, realizing how miserable I was studying Spanish, finally supported my decision to apply to culinary school. "Cooking seems like the one thing that makes you happy these days," my father admitted.

At the age of twenty, I dropped out of graduate school and gave up a full scholarship. Eagerly, I set my sights on the same school Julia Child attended and filled out the paperwork to attend Le Cordon Bleu in London. Within six months, I was on an airplane, leaving behind one course of study for another. Instead of analyzing texts and translating my thoughts into Spanish, I would be studying ingredients and creating works of art with food.

The program was a yearlong study of classical French cuisine. Initially I enrolled in the basic course to learn the fundamentals of savory food, but I quickly fell in love with the sweet side of dessert making. I added an additional program to master classical French patisserie, which doubled the time I spent in class each day. Mornings were spent observing demonstrations of classics such as *blanquette de veau*, beef consommé, and *Gateaux St. Honoré*. Afternoons I fastidiously followed my notes and attempted to reproduce each recipe in the allotted time for practicum class.

Coming from an academic background put me at a disadvantage to the other students in my class who honed their skills in the classroom of London restaurant kitchens. Their speed, agility, and finesses with ingredients far outmatched the clumsiness of my inexperienced hands in cooking. Still, what I lacked in culinary prowess I made up for in sheer intelligence and drive. I invested in an unwieldy copy of *Larousse Gastronomique*, the equivalent of the bible of French cuisine, and I cross-referenced my class notes until I had all but memorized each recipe for class. I created a system for time management so I could organize myself for success before each practical application.

Even though I began the year coming in dead last in execution and timeliness of recipe creation, I ended at the top of my cohort. I was chosen as lead pastry cook at our graduating class dinner for friends and family, which is an honor awarded by faculty to the student who shows the most promise in patisserie.

I graduated from Le Cordon Bleu at the end of that year with the Grande Diplôme, the coveted dual degree in French cuisine and patisserie. By that point, my credentials as a chef spoke for themselves. Following culinary school, I moved back to the United States and spent several years working stints in fine dining at The Ritz Carlton before becoming a sous chef.

My career followed a simple trajectory. I learned to cook the food I loved to eat. I left the restaurant business for that very same reason. I reached a point where the intensity of the work as a sous chef interfered with my ability to enjoy the food I prepared. Being around food was not the same thing as having the time to enjoy it. I missed the comfort of eating and was desperate for some relief. I believed at the time that private chef work was the answer. I could cook the food I loved and have the money and time to experience the best restaurants.

When I interviewed for my first job as a private chef at the age of twenty-five, the connection to my future employer was so immediate that I felt a sense of coming home. Not because of his multimillion-dollar home, or the Bentleys that lined the driveway, but because we spoke the same love language. We debated the quality of French Valrhona chocolate compared to the Belgian Callebaut. I understood his need for me to drive between the outer boroughs of New York to purchase a specific hand-rolled mozzarella, imported olive oil, and a fennel pork sausage from different Italian shops.

The job seemed idyllic—a food lover's dream come true, and a chef's carte blanche.

And it was . . . for a time. I rose every morning at six to make the same breakfast for my boss every day: two scrambled eggs with two pieces of crisp bacon. I had the next ten hours before dinner to shop and cook leisurely. As the Illy coffee percolated on the Carrara marble countertop, I combed through one of the hundreds of cookbooks that lined the kitchen's library. While my employer often dictated the main course for dinner that evening, such as his mother's recipe for veal cutlets or maybe chicken Scarpiello, desserts and sides were my choice. His one request was for one pure chocolate option and one non-chocolate. Pure meant that there could not be even a single fresh raspberry adorning a flourless chocolate cake or a hazelnut filling. It needed to be chocolate through and through.

That was for my boss, the foodie. He loved chocolate and wanted to taste the nuances in a particular variety. His wife was the opposite, and the non-chocolate dessert was for her. Her favorite was a dense almond torte flavored with a kiss of lemon zest. Usually, though, her desserts lay untouched.

By the end of this job, I was at my heaviest weight. My employer's rule was that he did not eat leftovers, so all the homemade pasta, luscious cheesecake, and extra helpings of chocolate mousse headed straight down to the living quarters I shared with the family's nanny. Along with several glasses of wine each night, we gorged ourselves on one decadent feast after another. The best ingredients New York had to offer, all prepared by a gourmet chef.

In the beginning, it felt like a fantasy. The money was alluring, and then there was the pleasure from all that food. Toward the end of my gig with this family, I had an annual physical with a doctor in town. It was the first time I had weighed myself in at least a year. The scale topped off at 185, and what I remember most from that visit was the doctor's unmistakable look of surprise at that number. On my 5'8" frame, I was a good thirty pounds heavier than my natural weight in high school.

"You need to watch your weight," he told me, not mincing words. It was the first and last time a doctor would ever be that straightforward with me. I gulped, embarrassed. Then, when the visit ended, I drove to Stone Cold Creamery and ordered a large mud pie mojo—coffee ice cream, Oreos, fudge, almonds, and peanut butter. *I'll start losing weight tomorrow*, I thought.

The report from the doctor coincided with my decision to leave the private chef position. I moved to DC to live with my parents while I searched for another opportunity, and I decided to stop hiding from the reality of my weight. My mother was an expert at calorie counting, so I decided to adopt her approach.

The process of learning to deplete my caloric intake so drastically was painstaking, as was using sheer willpower to deal with the intense hunger. Most people experience cravings, but the temptations are constant for a food lover who thinks, dreams, and lives for food. Even when I wasn't hungry, my brain offered a tantalizing feed of suggestions to eat. I pictured the perfect Moroccan chicken, studded with golden raisins, green olives, and the perfect blend of spice. I imagined how I would prepare it. Or I scoured the Wednesday edition of the *New York Times* and made a mental note of a new bakery that sold the best cinnamon buns the critic ever tasted. While I nibbled away at my low-fat turkey and lettuce roll-up, I eagerly devoured written recipes with my eyes, hoping to replace some of the pleasure I so desperately missed from my twelve hundred-calorie-a-day regime.

This began a decade of hills and valleys. Weeks of chicken breast and broccoli, sometimes half a cup of cottage cheese mixed with corn and black bean salsa. For a while, I dabbled in SlimFast shakes. No wine, no dessert, and at least thirty minutes of running, five days a week. I felt successful because I had figured out a system that took the weight off. What I didn't know was how to sustain it. All the while, my desire for good food simmered on the back burner, smoldering.

I couldn't snuff out my desire for food with willpower. Suggestions for bites, licks, and tastes still swirled around my mind, beckoning me. By the time I reached my goal weight, which was usually 155, I had my celebratory meal planned out. One thing was certain. There would be no deli meat or celery in sight.

I was in my late twenties, and between regular spin classes at the gym and adhering to a low-calorie diet on weekdays, I could offset weekend cheat days without regaining all those hard-earned pounds. I settled into another position working as a private chef for a new family, and this job allowed me to live independently. I was able to cook for this new employer without the added temptation of consuming any of the leftovers. The separation between work and personal life was clearly delineated.

A few years after starting this job, I met my husband, Alex. Within a year of marrying, we knew we wanted to start a family. My priorities began to shift. I was not willing to put the care and attention of my employer's family above my own, so I made the easy decision to leave my job as a private chef.

During my first pregnancy, I reveled in the expansiveness of each day without work. Alex left the house early, and I enjoyed the chance to wake up leisurely around 9:00 a.m. Between watching episodes of *No Reservations* with Anthony Bourdain or Rachel Ray's thirty-minute meals, I plotted what I would cook for myself that day. I was pregnant, after all, so nothing was off the table. I unashamedly baked and devoured homemade layer cakes, slow-cooked double-chocolate pudding with vanilla bean whipped cream, and lasagna layered with whole-milk ricotta and nubs of spicy pork sausage. It was gluttony at its finest.

I gained more than seventy pounds, and in pictures of me leaving for the hospital the night my son was born, I look like a well-stuffed Michelin Man. Pregnancy was my excuse to abandon any fear around gaining weight and give into every whim to eat. But once my first son was born, my body was something to be reckoned with. I felt like a balloon waiting to pop.

I didn't want to wear elastic pregnancy jeans for the rest of my life, so I talked Alex into buying a treadmill and then promptly started a strict, calorie-restricted diet. Hard-boiled eggs, a few slices of turkey deli meat, and raw broccoli with lite Ranch dressing was a rude awakening compared to the glory days of pregnancy. I suffered through it and doggedly ran in the basement on our new treadmill during my son's nap time. After about six months, I had lost most of the weight. I was in my early thirties, and it was not the first time I had to deprive myself to lose weight.

Enter forty: a decade loaded with meaning, especially for women. I had three healthy little boys running around at my feet, full of joy and plenty of energy. I had a supportive husband who loved me at any size and provided a substantial income to our growing family. And I was at home raising our children. It was the life I had always wanted.

When a low-level depression hovered and followed me around each day, there was no apparent cause. Paralyzing panic hit me, too, from time to time. I thought both were hereditary, not realizing until much later that they stemmed from overeating and drinking. Five o'clock was the magic hour. Kids were home, energy was up again in the house, and dinner needed fixing. Backpacks and shoes dropped to the floor, and I made a beeline to the fridge to uncork a bottle of Sauvignon Blanc. Standing at the kitchen island with that first glass, I could feel the tension in my shoulders soften and my mood started to lighten. It seemed that cocktail hour was always the solution to feeling better.

It was part of the natural rhythm of cooking for the kids in the evening, along with nibbles of nuts, chips, or the stray piece of cheese as the ingredients for a meal came together. One glass led to two or three, and my inhibition waned as I dished out and ate my supper alongside three little boys. Dessert was a yes, especially if I remembered to stock the pantry with my favorite ten-dollar jar of gourmet hot fudge and a stash of salted caramel ice cream in the freezer. I happily indulged during those two hours between five and seven before the kids got ready for bed. Life felt nearly perfect if I had a glass of wine in one hand and a spoon in the other. I crawled into bed most nights around 8:30, mildly comatose from the alcohol and dessert. I was never uncontrollably drunk, just pleasantly tipsy in a way that masqueraded as joy.

The buzz was short-lived, with a rude awakening on the other side of it. Around two in the morning, my eyes would blink open, wide awake. Acid churned in my stomach, beads of sweat lined the back of my neck, and sometimes I needed to walk around for several minutes to dislodge the internal gas before climbing back under the covers. It could then be another two hours before I fell back into any slumber. During that purgatory of sleeplessness, I wrestled with negativity. I was filled with thoughts of being a bad mom, resentment toward myself that I could not control my appetite, and generalized anxiety. The physical and mental anguish usually ended the same way, with me vowing to clean up my diet.

That was the start of most days in my early forties. By 7:00 a.m., I dragged myself out of bed to get the kids ready for school and guzzled down three cups of coffee just to cut through the brain fog. By 3:00 p.m., I was in the carpool line or slogging through DC traffic to pick the boys up from their different schools. By four, I was ready to unwind. Like clockwork, I started anticipating wine time.

***

This was my food story. It was a story of emotional hunger, and my love affair with eating and drinking that turned toxic. It began innocently enough, with food being the sixth love language in a family of food lovers. It evolved into a pursuit of pleasure, with food and wine being the suitor and me the damsel in distress.

Food was always there, waiting for me. I followed it everywhere, even to London for culinary school. There I discovered proper chocolate mousse is made with heavy cream and eggs, and that *Gateau St. Honoré* is a towering confection of cream puffs painstakingly dipped in hot caramel. Food was a labor of love. It led me back to the United States where I worked in fine dining restaurants, perfecting the slow method of risotto, each rice kernel growing creamier with the stir of a wooden spoon.

Food brought me to the homes of businessmen, where I diligently perfected their meals as a private chef. I drove through the boroughs of New York sourcing food, then recreating childhood recipes of my employer: veal cutlets, Manhattan clam chowder, and butterscotch pudding.

Finally, food brought me to my husband, whom I decided was the most important person, other than myself, to cook for. On our first Valentine's Day together, I surprised him with the ultimate gift—a six-course, homemade dinner paired with wine. We still talk about the chilled lobster and passionfruit salad, and the grapefruit sorbet intermezzo.

By the time I turned thirty, I still believed food was the one thing I had just for me. When I became a parent to my own three children, I relished my late-afternoon snack before school pickup. I found relief in cheese and crackers as I made dinner. And a bowl of chocolate marshmallow ice cream always took the edge off a long day.

Food was easy. Food was a pleasure. And my desire for it never ceased. In between meals, I devoured cooking shows and plotted what I would prepare for dinner. I read cookbooks as if they were novels, fantasizing about how the ingredients would manifest on a plate and taste on my tongue. I read restaurant reviews as if they were the daily news.

Fantasizing about the taste of my favorite pizza, perusing food blogs or restaurant websites, and using my free time to check out a new bakery in town were all ways I would use my mental energy during the day. When I entertained thoughts about food, they were like kindling to the flame of my desire to eat. The rush of dopamine in my brain from a slice of walnut-studded carrot cake after lunch quelled that fiery urge, but it also reinforced a pattern. The more I focused on food and obeyed momentary urges to eat, the more my brain was rewarded with the feel-good effect of dopamine. In the absence of reasoning from my higher brain, I would keep circling back for more pleasure from food.

There wasn't time for much else. I cooked; I ate. It was never enough. I could not find the stop button. Food was just too good.

But food could never rescue me from myself, and the longer I turned to it for relief, the worse I felt. The more I escaped the reality of my own life by eating and drinking, the more lost I felt—until one day I could no longer deny what I needed most.

Do you see yourself in my story? Perhaps your relationship with food looks different. But tracing the roots of your own love language with food is a necessary start to untangle the habit of overeating. To decode your emotional appetite, you need to first understand the role food played in your earliest memories. Spend some time reflecting on the following questions.

Food for Thought

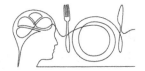

1. What are some of your fondest memories of eating as a child?
2. What was your parents' philosophy when it came to eating and drinking?
3. What role did food play in terms of nourishment, rewards, entertainment, connection, and relaxation?
4. How would you describe your personal relationship with food?
5. What boundaries, if any, were placed around food in your childhood home?
6. What did you learn about your body and the role of food in your own health?
7. When did you find yourself drawn to eating outside of daily meals?

Chapter 2:

The Tipping Point of Discomfort

By the time I was in my early forties, I could no longer ignore the downside of my love affair with food. After two glasses of wine, my energy felt zapped. During our usual Saturday evening movie time as a family, you'd find me dozing on the couch ten minutes into the show. I also noticed an uptick in urges to eat, and after drinking, I might negotiate a bowl of ice cream for myself from a less intentional place of reasoning. With a belly full of dessert and wine, it was hard to enjoy the pleasure of reading before bed since all I felt like doing was crawling under the sheets until morning. Yet my ability to sleep deeply always felt stifled by alcohol. I might easily drift off for the first few hours, but I always awakened to a restless feeling of anxiousness and indigestion.

Lying awake in the middle of night jolted my awareness. There is nothing like a 2:00 a.m. wake-up call to give you a perspective on life, and wine-drinking evenings always offered the same message: *This doesn't feel good.*

My intuitive sense liked to surface in that quiet space of darkness when none of the usual distractions of work or family could compete with it. It spoke softly but firmly and advocated for the truth to be heard. Unlike the urgent, spontaneous part of my brain, my intuition never demanded anything from me. It served as a compass, always guiding me back to what felt authentic and true for my best self. When I regularly drank, my voice of intuition was by my side in those midnight hours, often reminding me in a gentle way, *This isn't working for us.*

When I made the decision four years ago to change my relationship with food and wine, it was because giving into every impulse to eat and drink eventually made life less satisfying. The pleasure of food diminished the more I ate, and drinking beyond a certain point affected my sleep, mood, and energy. The consequences of being spontaneous every day were anything but fun. My impulses continued to lead me down the same path, and that path wasn't toward a richer, more fulfilling life. I was full of food and wine, and seeking more resulted in less of what I wanted out of life.

I was thirty pounds overweight with chronic indigestion and a stomach ulcer. I slept fitfully and depended on a nap every afternoon before I picked the kids up. A low-level depression descended, for no apparent reason, and I walked through each day in a brain fog.

One afternoon, I caught myself zoning out on the couch before dinner with a bowl of popcorn and a glass of Cabernet while the kids watched television in the background. It was a moment of awareness. This was not how I wanted to feel. I was looking for more than the bottom of an empty glass of Cabernet or the pint of coffee ice cream scraped clean by a spoon. In the moment, I thought I deserved it, when it came to the next delicious bite. Yet the aftermath of discomfort helped me realize that I deserved something more. I looked around at my life, full of blessings and abundant in things to eat and drink, and I still felt empty.

Choosing spontaneity and ease and pursuing pleasure from food and wine brought me down a dead end. I felt stuck. My identity revolved around food, yet the more I ate and drank, the more lost I felt. Somewhere along the way, in each spontaneous choice to indulge, I lost the plot of my own life.

When Food Becomes All-Consuming

I could tell that my habits with food and wine were paying the price on my body, but I felt like I had little control to change them. Emotionally, I felt my worst. I didn't think of myself as an emotional eater; I just believed I loved food too much. Back then I didn't connect the fact that "love" is the emotion of desire. I was so disconnected from my feelings because I spent most of my mental and physical energy chasing after the next delicious bite. I never gave myself the chance to stop and listen to what was happening inside of me.

It's hard to be in a good mood when you feel so physically unwell. What was obvious to me back then was how unhappy I felt. My body was rebelling against all the extra food and wine, and my emotional wellness could no longer be denied.

I was conflicted. How does someone who is passionate about food magically learn to stay in control and keep the weight off? I felt powerless—like there was a magnet pulling me toward that extra helping. Yet the misery I felt was unavoidable and begged for change. It was at this breaking point that I reached bottom. I needed a lifeline, and it wasn't going to come in the form of another diet.

I knew from previous experience that diets were part of the vicious cycle, not an actual means to an end. Following pre-scribed weight-loss plans only led me to obsess about food even more as I tracked, weighed, and calculated the right and wrong foods on the list. Feeling restricted to a diet was a recipe for overindulging and experiencing more helplessness. I couldn't go back for another round of being strict with myself only to fail miserably by regaining the weight.

I also wrestled with my identity and who I would be if I wasn't always turning to food. People knew me as "the chef." It was often the first way my husband introduced me to col-leagues. "Molly trained at Le Cordon Bleu," he would tell people. Friends called or emailed to tell me about a restaurant or ask for recipe advice. I had created a life that revolved around eating. That identity was eating me alive, but I also couldn't imagine parting with it.

I still felt passionate about food, but I was paying a hefty price to maintain my love affair with it. Not just the burden of physical pounds, but the way it consumed me physically, men-tally, and spiritually. It was the root of my dissatisfaction with life and how I showed up every day as a wife, mother, and forty-year-old woman in the prime of her life.

I focused intensely on food; it was all-consuming. I falsely believed it was my identity. Fortunately, food was never able to smother my spirit. Deep in the recesses of my soul, the truth slowly bubbled to the surface.

Somewhere in my body, a voice was rising. I believe there is a personal truth within each of us advocating for well-being. Some call it a conscience, others spirit. It's an intuition deep down that wants you to become the best version of yourself. It is the truth of your full potential.

While I felt conflicted about my desire for food and my need to feel better, I was not resigned. Something had been nudging me for years, deep within, to quit my daily wine habit. I also realized I was wasting my time on food, and it wasn't worth it. My mind was searching for an answer. I was open to finding a better way. I didn't yet know what it was, but I began listening for it.

I wanted a better path for my children, too. I didn't want them to believe food was the answer to their problems. I didn't want them growing up in a home where their parents poured a glass of wine like clockwork at 5:00 p.m. My three growing boys needed nourishment, but I also wanted them to understand their feelings and manage stress naturally. They needed to learn the difference between food as fuel and food as entertainment— what it means to feel energized by food instead of bogged down. I wanted them to be aware of how and what they consume.

There is no getting away from the social norms of our culture that value food to show love, celebrate, and socialize. Cupcakes, turkey dinners, and movie popcorn are some of life's momentary pleasures. I wanted to experience that along with my children. I wanted to sit down to a five-course dinner paired with wine in a fine dining restaurant from time to time. I didn't want to sacrifice my love of food, but I also wanted my kids to have a healthier relationship with it.

When I think back to that weekday evening on my couch at home, the boys watching TV in the background and me cradling a stemless glass filled generously with wine, I had two things on my mind. These two things are why I decided to act and why I couldn't wait any longer. They were my urgent reasons for not giving up.

1. I deserve to feel better at my age.
2. I want to show up better as a mom.

These two compelling reasons to change conflicted with my emotional appetite for food and wine. The more I followed that impulsive desire for the next bite, the less I showed up as the best version of myself. When I focused more on food instead of what my body needed to feel good, my health and well-being suffered. Pursuing a love affair with food, from an emotional instead of physical appetite, was counterproductive to my goals.

This is usually the case. Rewarding spontaneous urges for a quick hit of pleasure reinforces habits that undermine our ability to be our best. Our emotional appetite grows in response to the rate we give in to momentary desire and can detract from our long-term well-being.

But the body always tells the truth. For me, there was no denying how I felt, both physically and spiritually. It was the unmistakable voice of my intuition and the persistent pain in my body that eventually offset my desire for more food.

When I started paying more attention to my body and less to food, I moved closer to the truth of myself. I became interested in truly feeling better and began looking and listening for a solution.

One afternoon, I was driving in the car and listening to a podcast. Brooke Castillo, the popular life coach, asked, "If I could take away all your desire for food, would you let me?" Something inside me was intrigued. I was not ready to give up my beloved relationship with food, but I certainly wanted to desire it less. I needed the grip to loosen its hold over me. I longed for breathing room to think about other things and give my body a chance to heal.

My thoughts about food were endless—that it's irresistible, that it beckons me, that it's my life's calling. For so long, I called food my passion in life. I identified myself with it inextricably. That afternoon was a moment of awareness. Food is none of those things. It just sits there on a plate, lifeless. It's completely neutral.

It doesn't call my name or force its way down my throat. It doesn't tempt or taunt me or seduce me so that I can't say no. Food is not a lover waiting for me behind some dark corner in the kitchen, where nobody can see us. It doesn't wait for me or push its way onto my fork.

Food doesn't care about me one bit.

My problem with overeating and struggle with weight loss had nothing to do with food. But it had everything to do with my thoughts. This revelation took me a minute to digest. How could my ability to lose weight have nothing to do with food? During all those past years of dieting, I erroneously believed that focusing on the "right" foods was the solution to weight loss. That I just needed to distract myself from bad food choices and narrow my eating to virtuous foods. It dawned on me that dieting was only a way of shifting from one food obsession to another. Both avenues revolved around food and eating, so no wonder they perpetuated a cycle of consuming more than my body needed.

When I heard Brooke Castillo say on that podcast that "food is not the problem, your thoughts are," it was like someone handed me the key to a lock I had never been able to open. I could sense my inner truth, that voice I listened to more often these days, physically sigh with relief. It was like a pressing weight resting on my shoulders subtly lifted, and I felt instantly lighter.

There was hope.

It made sense to me in that moment that eating too much had less to do with food tasting good, and more to do with the reasons I ate that much food in the first place. It had to do with why I craved food when I wasn't even physically hungry. I now describe these reasons for turning to food out of pure desire as my *emotional appetite*. Unlike my physical appetite (which is noticed by typical sensations of hunger like growling, emptiness, and gnawing in my stomach) my emotional appetite is marked by any craving to eat when there was no physical hunger present.

The more I turned to food when my body didn't physically need nourishment, the more of a habit it became. My emotional appetite grew larger the more I responded to it with food.

Reflecting on my habitual patterns of eating, I knew that snacking provided an escape for me after a long day of managing my children. It was a way I connected with my family when we shared meals around a communal table. I comforted myself with food when I felt alone or frustrated. I also deprived myself of food I love when I believed it was the only way to offset overeating. I used food as the way to add pleasure, avoid pain, and take care of myself in the only way I knew how at that time.

When I discovered that food was not the problem, that it was really a matter of understanding my mindset and desire to eat, I immediately felt more empowered. The idea clicked as the missing piece of the puzzle in my journey to feel and look healthy. No previous diet, detox, or box of shakes ever addressed my desire to eat or why I overindulged. It was the reason they all failed in the long term. Temporarily, they were a quick fix. But eventually, willpower fizzled out, and the urgency for all my favorite foods kicked back in.

I knew that day that if I could learn to handle my thoughts about food and change my mindset around eating, I could lose the weight I needed and maybe even maintain it. I might even discover the freedom to eat the foods I love in moderation. I could feel in control around food, rather than at the mercy of every scrumptious morsel.

That day I embarked on a journey to change how I thought about my relationship with myself and food. It began with being open to something other than a conventional diet, and with believing I deserved to feel better. Instead of choosing to stay stuck in the habit of turning to food, I decided on behalf of my future self and what I believed was possible.

Changing my relationship with food turned out to be more about changing my relationship with *me*. I began the loving process of taking care of myself in a way I had never experienced with traditional diets. By showing up every day, even after a night of overeating, and honoring the commitment I made, I built trust with myself.

For a long time, it felt like my passion for food was an all-consuming relationship.

The price was too high. I discovered that no amount of creative inspiration in the kitchen resulted in any lasting satisfaction. And when I reached a certain age, the adverse effects of overeating often left me feeling physically and emotionally unwell. I was always one taste away from the next hit of flavor, delectable texture, or sweet sugar rush. On the other side of each satisfying morsel, though, was a deeper void that was not being satiated by food.

Yes, food kept me alive. But my over-desire for it never yielded the ultimate reward I hoped it would. Feasting was never the answer. Eating was simply a form of conditioning. It was the way I learned to navigate my life from a young age, a process of self-soothing. It propelled me down the line of a professional kitchen and helped me feel connected to home while I worked over every holiday.

I had to end my unhealthy pursuit of food to discover what I really needed most. I had to release the expectation that joy could be found outside of myself, in the next delicious nibble.

I started searching for contentment in the only place where I could truly find it: within myself.

These days, my old friend food still hangs around. But I no longer follow it. I let it do its own thing. And I, now, do mine.

I'm inviting you, dear reader, to start this journey for yourself. The rest of this book will take you down the path I followed to create an experience of freedom around food. I will guide you through the process of unraveling your emotional appetite and rediscovering your authentic self. You will learn how to separate your hunger to eat from your hunger for well-being, and what it's like to balance pleasure from food with pleasure in your body.

What I wish I knew back then is the secret I'll share with you now. As a food lover, you can learn how to enjoy food, and your body even more, with just a little sprinkle of awareness. Come with me as I reveal to you how to shift from mindless eating to mindfully connecting to your body.

What I've noticed through my own journey of eating and drinking less than I need is that it becomes harder to deny the truth of your body the more you start paying attention. Paying attention and developing that awareness is key.

The Tipping Point of Discomfort

Most of my clients reach a tipping point when the state of discomfort in themselves exceeds their desire to keep things easy and convenient. No amount of food or alcohol can repress their intuitive need for change. When people come to me for help in my business, it's because the discomfort of their physical experience outweighs the pleasure they get from eating.

Even though the idea of having another helping at dinner sounds convincing in the moment, the reality of what it feels like when they're bloated and uncomfortable afterward can no

longer be ignored. Or as much as they craved that slice of chocolate cake before bed, experiencing indigestion and restlessness
as they sleep overrides the momentary bliss they got from biting
into the dessert.

As we get older, it's often the case that our bodies are less
resilient to the effects of excess eating. Another way to think
about it is that our bodies become more sensitized to what we
need and what we can tolerate. I think this is a beautiful thing,
because through physical and emotional signals, your body is
giving you important information. Through feedback such as
insomnia, indigestion, lethargy, irritability, pain, energy, and
focus (to name a few), we can interpret what is truly serving us
and what is not.

What experience is eating creating for you right now? What
are you noticing? Start telling yourself the truth about it. Bring
consciousness back to the eating experience and back to your
body by paying attention.

There is delight in putting something delicious into your
mouth. But how delightful? What do you notice about the flavor,
texture, temperature, and overall mouthfeel of what you're tasting? When does that pleasure begin to fade?

In addition to reaching the tipping point of discomfort, most
of us also have at least one compelling reason to change that is
more important to them than the short-term pleasure of food. For
me, those reasons were (1) wanting a higher quality of life for
myself and (2) wanting to show up better as a mom.

Once I reached the tipping point of discomfort and had my
compelling reasons to change, I was ready to act. The next thing
I needed to figure out was the first best step.

Food for Thought

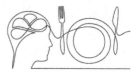

1. What is your body telling you these days about the impact of your current eating?
2. How would you describe the truth of your experience with eating and your intuitive sense about how well it is working for you?
3. In an ideal world, what would your ideal relationship with food and your body look like?
4. If you want to change how you eat, what is your compelling reason to do this? What is more important to you than the short-term pleasure of food?

Chapter 3:

The Why versus the How

L ife coaching taught me it was possible to feel completely empowered around food and helped me believe I could easily reach and maintain my ideal weight. In the beginning I wanted step-by-step instructions for how to do it. I was used to the methodical formula of a diet, and I assumed it was a matter of following the perfect process. But life coaching emphasized it was far more important to learn the reasons *why* I was overeating than it was for me to know *how* to eat less and lose weight.

It turns out that the *how* is far less important than the *why*.

I started to wonder, *If I'm not physically hungry, why am I eating? What role is food playing here if it's not for physical nourishment?* Before I changed my relationship with food, it felt familiar to eat more than my body needed, and it was easy to keep doing it. I was more focused on food and less on my body. I was used to looking outside myself for the solution. For many years, I thought the answer could be found in the next popular diet. But those approaches never worked because they only addressed the symptom of weight gain, not the cause of the overeating. They focused on *how* rather than *why*.

The old approach of dieting had me following someone else's formula, as if by following their rules I could micromanage my body into being the shape I wanted. Those rules had me believing there is perfect and right path for weight loss, as long as I didn't make any mistakes. One of the issues with the conventional rules of dieting is that many of us are inclined to rebel when someone tells us what to do. Since it's impossible to be perfect, it was easy for me to give up on following the rules, either by rebelling against myself or rewarding myself with food for a job well done. Because dieting keeps the focus on food and excludes the flexibility to fail and learn along the way, the result is an inevitable return to overeating. Following the rules of dieting actually increased my desire to eat and ultimately contributed to me gaining instead of losing weight.

These standard rules for weight loss are so widely accepted that for decades they informed my understanding of what it takes to feel and look your best. My diet mindset was so pervasive that even when I knew that dieting never worked long term, it felt hard to shake the old way of thinking. Staying fixated on those rules kept me from listening to my body and understanding the physical language of hunger, satiety, and emotions. It was tempting to keep returning to the old *how* of dieting, only because it felt familiar. But since I wanted different results, I needed to start with the *why* instead.

Old Rules of Dieting

1. There are good and bad foods.
2. Intermittent fasting is a quick-fix way to lose weight.
3. Exercise allows you to eat more.
4. Always stay within a calorie deficit.
5. Fat is bad.
6. No alcohol or sugar allowed.
7. You can splurge once a week on a cheat day.
8. Avoid tempting foods and banish them from the house.
9. Prevent hunger at all costs by eating throughout the day.

The Dance of Deprivation

When people focus on the how, they tend to have a restrictive relationship with food and deprive themselves on purpose. I'm not referring to people in impoverished situations who can't afford or don't have access to food. I'm also not including here individuals who eliminate certain foods for health reasons or because of physical sensitivities to those foods.

I'm talking about people, like my past self, who decide to avoid or give up foods they consider to be "bad," "unhealthy," or "too indulgent." Unconsciously, many of us have a belief around what's healthy and what's unhealthy, or the right and wrong way to eat for weight loss.

The dance of deprivation around food develops when someone believes they need to give up food they love to create the results they want. Feeling deprived is an emotional response to

believing that we can't have a particular type of food. Deprivation is not a factual circumstance, but rather a feeling created
based on a relationship with food. It's not a feeling that's particularly pleasant to experience, either. Many of us unknowingly fall into this dance of deprivation around food. It happens
when we believe we need to eat less than what satisfies our
body or when we believe we're not allowed to eat what everyone else is eating.

The experience of deprivation we create in our relationship
to food can be toxic. It always originates in our thoughts about
food. There is a difference between thinking, *I'm not allowed to
eat that*, and *I'm choosing not to eat this*. The former thought
implies that there is a rule in place, and we don't have permission to break it, while the latter suggests that we're fully empowered and in charge of our choices.

We are used to thinking there are either *good* or *bad* foods
to eat, or *right* or *wrong* ways to eat. This underlying "black or
white, all or nothing" thought process is one of the default patterns of our primitive brain, which we'll talk more about in the
next chapter. With the emphasis on low-calorie, low-fat, low-
carb rules for eating, old-school diets are built in a way that only
makes them practical for short-term, quick bursts of time.

In the absence of full fat, there is not only less flavor in food
but also the addition of additives that substitute sugar and artifi-
cial fillers for natural ingredients. Without fat, you feel less satiated by food and hungrier throughout the day. You sacrifice the
pleasure of taste and being satisfied physically and emotionally
from food. Natural, full fats have a minimal effect on insulin in
the bloodstream versus sugar and processed fillers that spike it.

This means your body is apt to burn fat rather than store it when you consume a moderate amount of full fat at meals.

Focusing on calories as your primary metric for meal planning and health is equally deceptive. A five-hundred-calorie bowl of chips compared to a five-hundred-calorie salad layered with veggies, protein, and a full-fat dressing has a dramatically different effect on your digestive system. The former choice, with very little nutritional value, will not only raise the insulin in your body and promote fat storage, but will leave you feeling underfed, lacking energy, and searching for more food. The salad, on the other hand, will provide nutrients to your entire body, satisfy your hunger, and increase your ability to focus and move throughout your day. Instead of increasing cravings for more food, having a meal balanced with carb-dense vegetables, satiating protein, and rich fat will lessen hunger and desire for more food.

Unlearning a diet mentality does not happen overnight. It begins by letting go of the idea that arriving at an ideal weight is the end goal. We are so used to treating the symptoms of our relationship with food instead of the underlying cause. The aim of this book is to help you identify why you turn to food beyond what your body needs, or why you deny yourself food in some instances. When you discover the reasons you overeat, you also learn more about your individual needs and what you desire. Getting more in touch with yourself and addressing these underlying needs makes overeating unnecessary.

When you resort to short-term, quick-fix tactics of the low-calorie, low-carb, low-fat variety, it stems from the belief that losing weight will solve the problem. That's why so many people are in a rush to reach their goal weight. There is a mistaken idea that changing your size will change the way you think and feel about yourself. It won't. A change in your physical appearance, without addressing the internal reasons that cause overeating, does not by itself create a sense of well-being or self-worth. It just creates a vicious cycle for most people who love food and don't understand how to manage their desire for it.

Still, many of us hold on to the idea that diets work.

Sometimes, during our initial consultation, a prospective client will tell me about a particular diet that works for them. They believe that when they follow the prescribed plan, they can lose the weight. I always reply to these statements with the same question. "If that plan works for you, why are you not doing it?" A plan is only as good as your ability to stick with it.

We usually rush through mainstream diets because they involve a lot of suffering. For most people, it's not doable long-term to eat a bland diet prohibitive of satisfying and flavorful ingredients. It requires sheer willpower to tolerate ongoing hunger and choke down chalky shakes that serve as substitutes for real food.

Willpower is not a reliable strategy for permanent results. The relentless determination to follow a strict way of eating will be exhausted within time, either when your results no longer seem worth the effort, or the unavoidable stress of life knocks you down. When this happens, after you've spent so much energy resisting the food you want, the repercussion has a boomerang effect. Your urge to eat bursts through the dam, and you're likely to make up for lost time by devouring everything you've missed out on. Regaining the lost weight is dispiriting, and you may even feel more discouraged than when you first began.

Still, you beat yourself up, believing you *should* be more disciplined. You fault yourself for not having enough self-control, being too disorganized, or just loving food too much. You turn it into a personal weakness that you can't maintain restrictive diets or find it hard to even commit to one. You often give up and fail ahead of time by not even trying.

You might fool yourself into believing that you just haven't found the "right" diet, and you cycle in and out of the latest trend, hoping there is a magic bullet approach you have yet to discover. I used to desperately wish that one day I would wake up, somewhere off in the future, and maintaining my ideal size would be effortless. I imagined that the frustration, humiliation, indigestion, guilt, shame, and agony would somehow disappear, like a magic trick, and erase itself over time.

It's even harder when you see other people eating what they want and losing weight. You fall into the trap of believing you're entitled to eat what you want and also be at your ideal size. Feeling entitled to food but not achieving the physical results you desire when you eat whatever you want makes it challenging to accept reality. Magical thinking around weight loss discounts the facts of what each individual person and their unique body need for a particular weight. Entitlement and wishful thinking only amplify the desire to eat more than what you physically need. This form of magical thinking fuels emotional eating.

There is also the fear of missing out to contend with in seeing other people eat food when you're not. Instead of recognizing your free will and agency in choosing what to eat or not eat, your mind naturally sees a chance to create the desire for food. Instinctual thinking of your primal brain will always be driven by the desire to increase pleasure, avoid pain, and conserve energy. So, without supervising your mind and creating a higher intention for yourself, you may fall prey to believing the side of you that wants instant gratification. What other people are eating and drinking is inconsequential to your body and how you feel and not a good indication of what you should be doing. But your brain is sneaky and will create a story entirely driven by trying to increase your chances of eating.

Your brain loves to use comparison as a default way of thinking about the world, other people, and the way things work. It's useful to gauge how things are done, acquire wisdom from other people's experiences, and decide what appeals to you. But often it turns into a way to disparage yourself and magnify the ways you fall short. Comparative thinking, when given free reign, will likely leave you feeling worse instead of better. It taps into another familiar thought habit of believing you're not good enough, you're inadequate, or you're less than other people.

Your brain believes that identifying inadequacy is helpful for long-term survival—as if by recognizing your shortcomings, you might address them and enhance your likelihood to be among the fittest. Yet the true result of thinking you're less than only discourages, instead of motivates, you to take action and see progress. Emotions associated with the thought *I'm not good enough* (and other variations of inadequacy thinking) are disempowering, and not the kinds of feelings that generate productive action.

It's useful to notice that nothing has gone wrong when your mind resorts to comparative thinking or points out your inadequacies. Remember, the brain is wired to do this. It's not a reason to be hard on yourself or add fuel to the fire of self-loathing. Your brain's negativity bias can easily lead you down a path of feeling completely incapable and broken if you let it. When you reach that place and are resigned to the idea that something is inherently wrong with you, there's a strong sense of powerlessness. Yet all along, your brain was simply left to its own devices.

Understanding the nature of your brain puts you in a position to accept yourself with compassion and be able to direct your thinking to serve you.

In my case, I mistakenly believed I loved food too much and would never have enough self-control to be at my ideal weight. At that point in my relationship with food, I depended on food and wine to feel better. It was the opposite of freedom.

What I discovered is that freedom around what I eat and drink happens when I feel empowered. When I have the confidence to trust myself around food and alcohol, I experience more peace and satisfaction. This kind of freedom, when I can handle desire for food and support myself emotionally without eating, creates a lightness independent of any number on the scale.

When I no longer needed food to escape myself, overeating became unnecessary.

Decoding the Scale

The scale is a useful tool for understanding feedback from the body as it relates to eating, but it can also be a source of agony if it's used the wrong way. Part of a conditioned diet mentality views the scale as a barometer of success and self-worth. My past self was tethered to the scale, hoping for that reward of the goal number, and it became a distraction from paying attention to the body. Sometimes I avoided the scale altogether because the negative thinking associated with seeing the wrong number was too painful to bear.

I had expectations for the scale that were heavy and daunting. How can a simple number carry so much emotional weight? Physical weight, displayed as a metric on a scale, is an important point of awareness. When mindless eating disconnects us from our body, the scale brings us back to it. It brings to light the truth of how our body is impacted by our habits with food. I felt shame around my physical weight when I believed the number on the scale determined my personal worth. Much of that is conditioned thinking, influenced by a society that values thinness. Once I discovered life coaching, I learned the advantage of using my conscious brain to change my inner dialogue and interpretation of weight.

To optimize how I felt in my body and develop confidence in my looks, the scale was an important ally. Instead of fearing it, I developed curiosity around it. I noticed the monthly pattern of my weight in response to the way I fed myself. When I took the focus off food and prescriptive eating, I was able to notice the relationship between my weight and how my body felt.

It's a big stumbling block when your weight doesn't match your idea of what you think you deserve to see on the scale. Realizing that what you eat and what you weigh on any single day is not always a direct correlation is useful in keeping your perspective in check. Remember, we're more interested in longevity and having a way of eating that can be maintained than immediate dips on the scale. The more you depend on the scale for gratification, the less likely you are to stay consistent. It's not only because your weight fluctuates for more reasons than just what you eat and the accumulation or disintegration of fat. Hormones, sleep, inflammation, illness, water retention, and stress are all viable factors that contribute to weight gain and may be totally unrelated to what you're eating.

Staying consistent is more likely when you deemphasize the importance of the scale and purposefully focus on other metrics of success. Weight loss is one piece of data that your way of eating may be giving you the results you want. But how does your body feel? When you discover the pleasure in your body with less food weighing you down, the desire to overeat diminishes. To make staying consistent easy, you need to cultivate a desire for feeling good above the pleasure of food.

The Difference between the Emotional and Physical Appetite

If I wanted to truly solve the issue and create permanent change, I knew I had to address the why instead of just the how. To begin to uncover the why, I needed to first identify the times I ate when I wasn't physically hungry. It started with the question, "Am I hungry?" and led to the question, "If I'm not hungry, why do I want to eat right now?" These questions turned the focus away from food and back to my body.

Making the decision to stop eating more than my body needed helped me see the difference between what I began to call my *emotional appetite* and my *physical appetite*. When I was stuck in the cycle of turning to food with every impulse to eat, the voice of my desire sounded much louder than the subtle language of my body. The more I responded to the desire to eat, the less aware I was of what my body needed. It became habitual to override what my body needed because the desire for food felt so strong.

Our *physical appetite* is the experience of hunger, or the voice of our body telling us it needs to be nourished. Our *emotional appetite* begins in our brain and stems from our thoughts. This thinking creates the emotion of desire in our body. Every time I continued to eat when I wasn't physically hungry, my emotional appetite increased.

When the reward center of the brain gets the dopamine surge from food, it goes to work on figuring out how to create more of that pleasure. The habit chain builds between thoughts, the feeling of desire, and the act of eating, and it locks into place the association between food and a particular situation. That's why, like clockwork, I had the urge to eat a snack at 3:00 p.m. every day before picking my kids up from school. I ate to relax and feel good during a typically stressful time of my day.

It never occurred to me to ask, "Am I hungry right now?" I was used to listening and answering to my emotional appetite which simply said, "I want that," or "This will make me feel better." When I committed to change the habit of overeating, I decided to pay attention to what my body was telling me. I realized that I couldn't remember the last time I'd felt true hunger pangs. I made the decision to eat in response to my body, whenever there was either growling, gnawing, or that empty pull I know now as physical hunger.

This simple shift was the beginning of turning my focus away from food and back toward my body. My physical appetite was the best indication of what I needed to feel nourished and energized. Along with the rumble of hunger, I also listened for the subtle whisper of satiety.

How did I know when my body had enough? I used to think that fullness, and the discomfort of being stuffed with food, was a sign I was ready to stop eating. But I realized that the weighted feeling I used to experience was a sign I'd had too much. Being satisfied and feeling full are two different sensations. The former quells hunger just enough while maintaining lightness in my body, while the latter feels more like being bogged down and heavy.

The more I listened to my body, the more I distinguished subtleties on the spectrum of hunger and satiety. I sensed the nuance between mild and prolonged hunger and determined a comfortable point when I could eat to satisfy that sensation without overfeeding myself. Once that hunger faded, I experimented with stopping at different points of satiety so I could observe how my body felt an hour or more after eating.

My physical appetite became clearer the more I connected to my body before, during, and after meals. It was a process of getting to know my own unique needs and how to optimize feeling my best. It was fascinating to relearn that my body knew exactly what it needed. My body wants to feel its best and sends me cues to help me understand what it needs. We are both on the same team and can support each other in creating the ideal relationship with food.

Along with physical cues, my body also communicated its emotional language. By taking the focus off food, I noticed all the sensations and vibrations making themselves known inside me. At times, the physical hunger I felt was layered with the skittish energy of urgency, and I observed how the quickening of that emotion changed the way I thought about my hunger.

My body was a foreign territory at the beginning of this journey, and I was discovering the entire landscape of physical and emotional needs. Its language felt foreign, but over time I learned to distinguish between the dialects of how it communicated with me. Instead of rejecting my body's physical and emotional expressions, I tried to accept and honor them. It was the beginning of building trust with myself and creating a sense of safety inside of me.

Learning how to listen to the language of my body took some practice, but over time it became a new habit. I remember one day at the beginning of my journey when I felt a strong urge to eat, and it had nothing to do with being physically hungry. I had applied for a job, and I believed I had all the ideal qualifications. It was a dream position, one that incorporated all the things I loved to do, and my application was strong. Yet I learned that someone else was chosen for the role. Immediately I felt a strong impulse to open a bottle of wine, pull out some chips, whip up some guacamole, and go to town on eating. I felt antsy, as my brain scanned all the delicious options available to me in the fridge. Like a GPS system, it pulled up a mental map of where the available treats were stashed and began populating my brain with suggestions of what to eat.

There were no pangs of physical hunger, just the fast, frenetic energy urgently willing me to get up and start scouring the kitchen. I remember being in my bedroom, taking a deep breath, reconnecting with my body. The emotional vibration of urgency was quick and strong, but when I relaxed into it, I got curious about the emotion underneath. I asked myself, "How are you feeling right now?"

I realized that I was dealing with disappointment or possibly frustration. When I acknowledged that these feelings were valid, I could accept myself in that moment and give myself permission to feel that way. The urgency layered on top of disappointment was my old habit of trying to feel better and using food to numb the vibration of my emotional state. My emotional appetite in that moment was urging me to seek food as a panacea—to escape the uncomfortable vibration of disappointment and frustration, and then the restless urgency. It dawned on me that I was experiencing multiple emotions at once, and it was a foreign experience to navigate and create space for each one.

Through my breathing, I dialed into where I felt the tension. I pictured the oxygen entering in through my nose, dropping down to the space inside my chest where the energy of disappointment resided. I pictured that same breath expanding the area and opening up my ability to feel disappointment and frustration for what they were. I imagined trying to explain to a doctor, in very physical terms, what it was like to experience these emotions. I felt a heavy weight in my chest, and as I breathed into it, pressure rose through my throat. The frustration even expanded into my head, and I noticed a pulsing sensation at the base of my skull.

The more I connected to my body and stayed curious about my emotions, the safer I felt experiencing these feelings. I realized that while they felt foreign and uncomfortable, they were not nearly as scary as I initially thought. I didn't need to escape the experience through eating. In fact, eating would not truly help me feel better. It would only add another source of tension to feeling disappointed and frustrated.

If food is no longer the way you numb and soothe the vibrations of anxiousness, boredom, frustration, or any other uncomfortable feeling, what do you do with those feelings instead? That, too, is part of the work of responding to the language of your body and becoming capable of managing your feelings. Many of us have never been taught how to handle our emotions, and eating becomes a convenient way to avoid them altogether. But processing your feelings instead of burying them with food creates peace of mind and personal fulfillment that no amount of food can ever provide.

Through understanding your unique emotional appetite, you'll get to know more about the role food plays in your life. You'll start to understand yourself better and what you need to be truly satisfied. By first comprehending why you eat beyond what your body needs, you can learn to solve those needs without the extra food. Those needs were never meant to be solved with food, anyway. Food just happens to be a convenient, delicious distraction.

Your desire to eat is far more complex than simply needing physical nourishment. When desire presents itself and is allowed the space to be present (without food pushing it down), you can consider what it is there to tell you. If food is not the answer, how would you satisfy that desire?

All your control lies in the present moment when you can identify and connect with your body in its physical and emotional language. When you witness what's happening emotionally in your body, you have the room to choose how to respond. Overeating is a way you try and make yourself feel better, instead of allowing yourself to feel uncomfortable at times. But why deliberately feel uncomfortable?

Because discomfort is inevitable. Even when you choose to overeat to avoid negative emotions, you're never really escaping the discomfort. You're just creating some temporary pleasure, and momentarily dulling the vibration of an emotion like anxiousness. Food gives you a slight distraction, or reprieve, from the anxiousness. But it doesn't resolve the anxiousness.

The negative emotion, whether it's anxiousness or something else, is still there in your body waiting to be processed. But now, by eating you've layered on the discomfort of feeding your body food it doesn't need along with the burden of extra digestion, lack of energy, guilt, indigestion, and weight gain. You went from having the discomfort of anxiousness to adding on the additional discomfort from the aftermath of eating. What's also worth recognizing is that now you've created a habit of turning to food for comfort and increased your desire for it. There is a level of discomfort in the extra mental chatter around food and the frequency of urges you contend with.

There is no path in life without discomfort, even though we perpetuate the idea in our thoughts and actions that we should always feel good, that we should be happy instead of sad. But it's the contrast of positive and negative feelings that creates a rich life experience. We are designed to experience negative feelings on purpose, and getting good at experiencing them can end the cycle of overeating. Which flavor of discomfort do you prefer to experience?

Even once you decide to change your relationship with food and practice being conscious, there might inevitably be times when you decide to overeat anyway. When this happens, you'll usually become conscious again when the physical symptoms of overeating kick in. You notice the new level of discomfort and recognize that more food will only make it worse. This used to happen to me in the middle of the night after a night of drinking. Consciousness felt like a rude awakening—like cold water being poured over my head.

When you have an experience like this, it can be easy to do one of two things: give yourself a hard time for it or dismiss it and try and forget it even happened. Neither of these options help you learn from the experience and continue evolving into the version of yourself you're striving for. Verbally chastising yourself from a place of guilt and shame only encourages more eating as a way of escaping how you feel. It keeps you stuck in a loop of feeling worse instead of better. Brushing off the experience, while maybe better than beating yourself up, also blocks your ability to stay conscious and understand what happened.

Rediscovering your internal needs and desires is the path to freedom. Knowing how to support yourself through emotional distress and fulfill your passion for a meaningful life is how you create a rich and satisfying life. Food cannot provide you with that, and neither can people you depend on. You are the source of your own misery, and the source of your own happiness.

In Part II, we'll take a deeper dive into what I call the spectrum of emotional appetites, the signature reasons why I and many of my clients developed the habit of overeating. As you read these stories, you may recognize your own.

But understanding why I depended so much on food all began with the decision to only eat when I was physically hungry and had planned to eat. This made it easier to recognize my emotional appetites in the first place.

This was a radically different approach from conventional diets I followed in the past. I used to think I needed to eat in a virtuous way, hit the gym multiple times, give up fat, drink detox shakes, use intermittent fasting, or have a splurge day once a week. It was a pervasive diet mentality that kept me returning to the yo-yo cycle of deprivation and regaining weight.

That's why understanding the why is more important than knowing the how. When you make sense of why you eat more than your body needs, the how begins to take care of itself. Addressing the source of the issue, while unfamiliar and potentially uncomfortable at first, helps clarify the solution and make the process a whole lot easier.

What your body wants is to be at its natural weight—to have energy and not be weighed down. To have mobility so you can feel invigorated by easily taking a walk and can release internalized stress naturally. To have strength so you can carry things throughout your day without injury. To have ease so you sleep soundly and feel rested and restored every day.

But as a food lover, it can be confusing when you have so much desire to eat.

It might seem like you have an insatiable appetite, or that your body needs more food.

But now you know that physical hunger and emotional hunger are two totally different things.

Wait a second, Molly, you're probably thinking, *I'm not an emotional eater. I just love food.*

I love food just as much as you do (maybe even more). What I discovered, though, after eating in excess for many years, is that love and desire for food are emotions, too. Wanting extra food, craving extra food, having the urge for more and more food—all these feelings are coming from your brain and your thoughts about food. When you tell yourself, night after night, that a bowl of popcorn and a glass of wine will help you unwind after the kids are in bed, you feel a desire for those things.

When your brain suggests that you need something crunchy as an afternoon snack and a break from work, and you believe it, the desire to eat kicks in. Or maybe it's the belief that a little something sweet is the perfect way to end a meal—and the craving for ice cream that follows it.

Notice how all these thoughts, when believed, generate a desire for food.

We underestimate how much our thinking elevates our desire for food and alcohol, because so many of our well-practiced thoughts just seem true. It's only because we've believed them for so long that they seem true.

This cycle of thoughts, emotions, and actions, when regularly connected, are easily repeated over and over again. I used to repeatedly tell myself how it was hard for me to resist ice cream and that I wasn't satisfied with only three scoops. It seemed almost like a fact that was true. Telling myself that thought repeatedly created the desire for ice cream.

You might identify yourself as someone who is a chocoholic, or you might say you have a sweet tooth in a matter-of-fact way, not realizing that every time you claim that belief, it resolidifies the desire for chocolate or sweets.

To eat in a way that aligns with your body feeling and looking its best, you need to listen more to the physical language of your body and less to the suggestions of your brain for food. Your body's signals—indigestion, fatigue, energy, focus, illness, hunger and pain—will bring you back to the truth of what you need. When you are in alignment with true hunger, you know it's time to eat. When you understand true hunger and your ideal satisfaction level for your natural weight, it's easy to stop at enough. Then you are in harmony with your body.

The act of overeating and the symptom of being overweight are both signs that you're out of sync with your body. They are signs that you're stuck in a habit, generated by your mind.

This is the best news in the world—because the only thing standing in your way between doing what your body wants and being at your ideal weight is changing the habit. Since habits begin and end with our thinking, you can't underestimate the role of mindset in your relationship with food and eating. On the other hand, when you go through the motions and follow a prescriptive diet, you only change the food without examining the thoughts driving the eating.

Now that we've covered the why, it's time to talk about the how. In the next few chapters, we look at the keys to creating conscious habits that result in lasting change. And it all begins with the brain.

Food for Thought

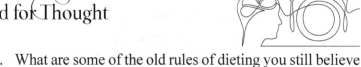

1. What are some of the old rules of dieting you still believe to be true?
2. If you could create new guidelines for caring for yourself, what would they be?
3. What are some rules of dieting you're ready to let go of and why?
4. What are some patterns you notice around the times you eat beyond hunger and satiety?
5. What are some reasons you turn to food when you don't need it for physical nourishment?

Chapter 4:

The Primitive and the Conscious Brain

Remember that I told you this would be a journey where all roads lead back to you? By identifying my compelling reasons to change and believing it was possible to change, I was ready to commit to change. Commitment began with this belief in myself. I learned, as I was introduced to life coaching, that thoughts about myself are the fuel for how I feel and act. Committing is often the hardest part, but the most necessary.

When I made the decision to act, I began to reclaim my authority over my body and my life. Instead of continuing to think I was powerless around food, I took ownership of how I felt and my ability to do something about it.

Making a commitment to myself created a sense of empowerment. It marked the beginning of experiencing freedom around food, but I still had a lot to learn to make it a permanent

63

change. One of the things I learned from my own coach was the power of making decisions ahead of time. My commitment to change my relationship with food and trust in the possibility that I could end the struggle was the first of these decisions. After so many years of pursuing the next delicious bite, I didn't trust myself to stop at a moderate portion. Making the first decision to commit to a new approach was the way I slowly began to rebuild that trust.

More than anything, I was curious whether it would work. I was intrigued by the idea that I could manage my cravings in a new way. I discovered, by learning more from my coach, the role of my thinking about food and how my thoughts played a role in the strong pull I felt toward food. But just because I knew what to do didn't mean I could easily do it. My old dieting habits of focusing on the food rather than why I wanted the food weren't simple to break. What I learned is that two parts of the brain are crucial in managing urges to eat. For the purposes of this book, I will call these two parts the *primitive brain* and the *conscious brain.*

Your Primitive Brain: Decoding the Habit of Overeating

The primitive part of the brain is instinctive in nature. It functions to keep us alive by anticipating danger, responding spontaneously, and urging us to seek comfort. This part of the brain is driven by the need to stay safe, keep things easy, and avoid pain. It motivates us to seek pleasure, because it's the opposite of pain and that must mean it's good for our survival. It also encourages us to expend the least amount of energy possible because if we are rested, there is a better chance we will thrive.

In prehistoric times, this survival mechanism of the brain served an important purpose, since everyday survival was less certain than it is now. These days, there aren't the same immediate threats, and we can survive independently more easily. Still, the primitive brain has not evolved beyond the needs of our earliest ancestors.

So, how is this relevant to the habit of overeating?

The way the primitive brain conserves energy and keeps things easy is by turning regular actions into *habits*. It takes usual patterns of thinking, feeling, and acting and routinizes them by storing them in the unconscious part of the brain. Also, since this part of the brain is motivated by pleasure, and food is a big source of that, it makes associations between situations when we eat and encourages us to do more of it through thoughts that create desire for food.

When I began learning about my brain and the role it plays in overeating, I discovered how the powerlessness I felt around food was just an ingrained habit.

The primitive brain is also home to the reward center of our minds. Pleasure is released in the brain through dopamine with things that create pleasure and perpetuate survival. Eating creates a dopamine reward, and that motivation encourages the primitive brain to seek more.

We are meant to desire food since it nourishes us and maintains health. But not all foods are created equal. Whole foods that come from the earth and are slowly digested by our bodies release a natural amount of dopamine, while processed foods that are refined and condensed from their original form create a more intense dopamine response.

It's the difference in your brain between eating an apple and a slice of chocolate cake.

Whole fruit, with its natural sugar and fiber, has a subtle, feel-good effect on the brain. Chocolate cake, made with processed flour and sugar, creates a more intense dopamine response in the primitive brain. The brain mistakenly assumes that this means chocolate cake is important for survival. It increases desire for it by suggesting thoughts that motivate the eating of it. Feeling a compulsive need for more chocolate cake and acting on this makes us feel worse instead of better in the long term. The primitive brain is confused about food.

The habit of overeating is driven by the primitive brain through thoughts like *I want that*, *It's my favorite*, *I don't want to miss out*, *I deserve this*, and many others. That thinking creates a desire and an urgency to eat even when we're not physically hungry. I learned that every time I gave into an urge and ate, the dopamine reward in my brain reinforced the thought, feeling, and action habit. The cycle of turning to food out of desire was more and more ingrained until the habit seemed uncontrollable.

Eating from urgency happens naturally because your brain connects the visual stimuli of food on a plate, or snacks on the counter, with desire to consume it. Unless, of course, it's food you dislike. Notice then how you might have zero interest in eating it. The only difference when there is food on the counter you dislike is the thought you have about it. One person can see chocolate and quickly feel a craving for it if chocolate is something they especially love, while someone else who might be allergic to chocolate has a completely different thought and emotional response to it. For the person who dislikes chocolate, there might be a complete lack of interest in eating it.

That's how powerful our thoughts are about food. When it comes to having the relationship you want with food and feeling empowered about how you eat it, your thoughts are everything. Your thoughts are within your control, and they are where all the power lies.

When your brain instinctively makes the connection between food you like and the desire to eat it, intentional thinking can change the response of reacting to that urgency. When you learn to develop some awareness around your emotions, you become familiar with what an urge feels like inside your body (which is distinct from physical hunger).

In my case, I notice my heart racing and a quickening in my energy. Sometimes my thoughts race, too, and it can feel like a desperate need to eat the food. If I'm hungry, and the food looks especially good, I can start feeling this way while I am grabbing the ingredients to begin cooking.

This might lead to an impulse to snatch bites and nibbles of what I'm preparing before the cooking is even finished. If you give into that initial craving to eat while you're cooking, it can seem even more challenging to stop yourself from continuing to graze. This is because once you reward the urge with food, two things happen that reinforce the habit. The first is that your brain gets a flood of dopamine from the food and strengthens the neural pathway between your thought *I want that*, the feeling of desire, and the reward in your brain. It's likely your brain will rely on that thought again and offer up more desire to eat when you're prepping food in the kitchen.

The second thing that perpetuates the habit of spontaneous eating is that once you get the taste and pleasure of food in your mouth, the desire for more intensifies. If you're like me, you might fall for the old thought *I'll just have one taste* before realizing that the first taste is what opens the floodgates of wanting more. That's not to say all is lost at that point and you should just give into all the justifications of your brain. Each moment is an opportunity to interrupt the pattern, and with some practice, you can feel even more confident doing this.

It's when the habit of overeating is so ingrained that it can feel impossible to stop yourself and exercise any form of self-control. But the same habit you created with those unconscious thoughts and feelings can be unraveled with some insight into what is happening and awareness around your regular patterns. Because the primitive brain is the oldest, most hardwired part of the brain, its thinking responds first and can sound the loudest. It's like a toddler, demanding its needs be met, and it throws a fit without some supervision. It might feel like the easiest thing to do is just give in and succumb to the demands of your brain. It may also seem like there is no other option. But the truth is, you're still entirely in charge.

Pay attention to the way your mind fantasizes about food to instigate a desire for it. You may notice yourself imagining the cookie and picturing going into the kitchen to eat it. This is your brain's way of visualizing something it wants before it happens. Picturing yourself buying or eating something in advance is a very subtle way that urges start to manifest in your brain. If you're not careful and not aware of what's happening in your mind, you may begin agreeing with the suggestion that a glass of wine or handful of chips would be a great idea before dinner.

Think of these initial fantasies as suggestions from your primitive brain, testing the water to see if you take the bait. It can seem as innocent as picturing yourself driving to a new pizza shop and ordering a slice of their meat lover's special. Maybe you came across an ad for it and your mind latched on to the idea that it would taste delicious. It's almost like you mentally create a plan of how you will get from your desk chair to the pizza parlor. Unconsciously, you might entertain the fantasy and unknowingly ratchet up your desire for the pizza. Before you know it, you've formulated a plan to pick up pizza later that afternoon.

When you unravel an experience of overeating like this, you'll see that there can be a chain reaction between a seemingly innocent suggestion from your brain to the act of overeating the food in the moment. The desire begins with your initial consent to entertain the idea of a particular food or beverage, however many days, weeks, or months in advance of you actually eating it. It might be as subtle as thinking, *It might be nice to have a glass of Pinot Noir one night*, without the realization that you've just ignited the flame of desire in your unconscious mind. Perhaps you buy your favorite bottle to have "on hand" or because it happens to be on sale—and ever so subtly, you've alerted your primitive brain.

Your Conscious Brain: The Path to Freedom

The part of your brain that can "pay attention" to what is happening, and even plan for it, is your *conscious brain*. Unlike the primitive brain, which is only responding to its antiquated reward system for survival, your conscious brain can think intentionally for long-term well-being. It thinks rationally of your best interest and strategizes to help you succeed at feeling your best.

Along with the conscious brain, your body reveals the truth of your choices around food. Your body is a sensitive system that's acutely aware of its physical needs. It alerts you through indigestion, fatigue, and general malaise (among other symptoms) that it does not respond favorably to certain foods. It also shows you through increased focus, energy, and positive mood that it feels better when it's properly nourished.

To change the habit of overeating, you need to engage your conscious brain more than your primitive brain and focus more on what your body is telling you.

When you use your conscious brain to rationalize, you start to learn the effect that eating in excess has on your body. Giving into the momentary impulse for more sugar leads to less pleasure over time and will lead to feeling worse. If you've been around children who ate too much sugar, you know there can be a state of frenzied energy followed by a crash and burn. Children who are given everything they demand tend to appreciate less and want more. Like the primitive brain, children are not thinking long term or about their best interest. It is up to the parent to impose boundaries and supervise what goes into their children's mouth, knowing that less sugar will lead to more well-being. When it comes to food, we need to parent ourselves using the higher part of our brains and think mindfully about how we want to feel in the future.

Supervising is different from enforcing. Parenting yourself around food means supporting yourself in how you want to feel holistically, not acting like a militant dictator policing every move. In the former instance, you are coming from love and your own best interest. In the latter, you are being punitive and likely to rebel against yourself. Using your conscious brain to think intentionally about your choices with food takes practice, but it enables you to regain control over your relationship with what goes into your mouth. The goal is not to eliminate pleasure or make food boring, but rather to enhance the overall pleasure you experience in life.

If you're someone who uses food as your primary source of pleasure, notice how you diminish the pleasure felt in every additional bite. Overeating for pleasure limits the pleasure felt in your body, the pleasure of your emotional health, the pleasure of utilizing your mind, and the pleasure of engaging deeply with others.

Where is pleasure felt? Our five senses are receptors, and when we eat, we engage all of them when we are being fully conscious. Yet mindless eating, done in response to a primitive impulse, is the opposite of conscious eating. It's reacting to a feeling, whether desire or disappointment, that leads us to eat to feel better. Reactive eating, instead of intentional eating, robs us of all the pleasure to be had from food.

Sometimes I hear clients say, "I don't want anyone telling me what to do, so I don't plan at all." This is allowing the primal part of your brain to run the show, which is essentially letting it *tell you what to do*. If you're satisfied with the results of always obeying the demands of your primal brain, there's no need to supervise it or question its patterns. Yet most people don't like the sense of helplessness, feeling out of control, and being at the mercy of urgent impulses around food. Your primal brain, when left to its own devices, will always make a beeline toward food and instant gratification. It's prioritizing dopamine, after all.

Many of us are not used to talking back to ourselves. If you're like me, you may not even realize you have the option. The voice of your primitive brain pipes in with its proclamations that sound like "We're just eating this today," "Who cares," and "It doesn't make a difference anyway." It seems like a decision has been made, and the easiest thing to do is comply. But who is making the decision? It's important to remember that whether you agree with your primal thinking and the demand for more food in the moment, or whether you respond intentionally with "That's not on the plan, so we are choosing not to have it," it's still *you* who makes the call.

It's empowering to know that you always have the final say. You always choose whether food makes it into your mouth.

Remember, supervising your primal brain doesn't need to be harsh, militant, or accusatory to be effective. Acknowledging when you want food that you may not need and kindly reminding yourself of your choice to not eat right then goes a long way to diffusing the tension. When your brain urges you, saying, "We need to have that cookie right now," you might try answering yourself with "I know you really want that right now, but we're choosing to wait until dinner to eat today."

We mentally relate food and drink boundaries with rules we must follow instead of simply choices we make ahead of time with intention. When there are rules involved that we "have to" follow, part of us naturally wants to rebel. Often, we think being spontaneous is more fun than planning meals in advance. Without premeditation, choices require less thought and deliberation, and on the surface that seems easier. Going with the flow, being unconstrained, and doing things spur-of-the-moment is not freedom around food, though. Think of the burden that comes with eating until you're stuffed, not being able to control yourself around food, and experiencing the guilt that sets in.

The truth is that when I gave my primitive brain free reign over choices around food and wine in the moment, I felt powerless. Without supervision, my mind always led me back to where it got the biggest, instantaneous reward. When you give your attention to food, and it becomes a main source of pleasure, you'll find that your thoughts and feelings motivate you to prioritize it above other things. My main source of pleasure was also the root of my discomfort. There was no escaping negative consequence of letting my primitive brain dictate my choices with food.

Fantasizing about the taste of my favorite pizza, perusing food blogs or restaurant websites, and using my free time to check out a new bakery in town are all ways I would use my mental energy during the day. When I entertained thoughts about food, they were like kindling to the flame of desire to eat. The rush of dopamine in my brain from a slice of walnut-studded carrot cake after lunch quelled that fiery urge, but it also reinforced a pattern. The more I focused on food and obeyed momentary urges to eat, the more my brain was rewarded with the feel-good effect of dopamine. In the absence of reasoning from my higher brain, I would keep circling back for more pleasure from food.

Spontaneity with food, while seemingly fun and easy in the moment, can establish a habit of overeating that feels difficult to control. It takes the thoughtfulness out of why you are eating and lessens your ability to thoroughly enjoy the food in your mouth. Instead of feeling satisfied, you might even feel disappointed, because most of the pleasure is lost in the mindless urgency to eat quickly. You're left with disappointment and the uncomfortable fullness in your body, and that can drive you to go back for even more.

This creates a tug-of-war in your mind between the pull of pleasure from food and the need to listen to your body. The loop of spontaneous thoughts, leading you back to more food, is very persuasive. But there is no mistaking the truth of your physical well-being. Your body keeps the final score.

Spontaneous choices around food, when left unchecked, lead to less freedom instead of more. Instead of feeling empowered in front of a buffet of your favorite foods, you feel out of control. You don't trust yourself to enjoy a little bit of a few things. You're frustrated that you continue to eat when you're clearly full. Mobility, getting dressed, sleeping well, and having the focus to get through your day all become harder.

Consciousness, not spontaneity, is the path to the life of your dreams, as we'll see in the next chapter.

Food for Thought

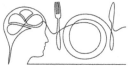

1. What are some of the reasons you give into spontaneous eating?

2. How would you describe the experience of spontaneous eating before, during, and after it happens?

3. What is the upside to eating mindlessly when you give into cravings for food?

4. What is the upside to making intentional choices with food and eating with awareness?

5. When you imagine experiencing full freedom around food, what comes to mind?

6. What is one small step you can take today to feel freer in your relationship with food?

Chapter 5:

From Mindless to Mindful Eating

Consciousness is the state of being fully present in the moment, utilizing our senses to bring awareness to the here and now. For me, it began with redirecting my focus away from food and back to my body. Honoring the cues of physical hunger, fullness, and emotional vibrations recentered me to where all my power lies. Food never had the authority over me, but when I let my primitive impulses take over, it was easy to feel disempowered. My process of unlearning the habit of mindless eating was a journey of developing awareness in my body, engaging my conscious brain, and responding less to those primitive reflexes.

Since the primitive brain is more spontaneous and habitual, utilizing the conscious brain requires thinking ahead of time to override momentary impulses. So, in my commitment to change the habit of overeating, I needed to engage my conscious brain to make fewer spontaneous choices with food and

more intentional ones. This involved planning the day before about what to eat.

My coach recommended that I make a boring food plan with foods I didn't love. She said if I wanted to lessen my desire to eat, I needed to stop looking forward to meals. While I resonated with everything she taught me about brain science, thoughts, and habits, it didn't jibe with me that I should get rid of my passion for food. I remember thinking, *If I need to choose between eating food I love and being in a body I love, I will choose food every time.*

My commitment waned at the idea that eating needed to be boring, so I decided to forge my own way. I leaned into the possibility that you could be a food lover and still be in your ideal body. In the first phase of unlearning the habit of overeating, I simply thought through my food choices ahead of time. I balanced what I knew about processed foods, and how they increase desire to eat more, with foods that both tasted good and felt good in my body. I imagined myself at my ideal weight, and I pictured not just a thinner frame, but someone with more energy and focus. Each night I made simple choices about what I would eat the next day, and I saw those choices as steps to becoming my future self.

The first iteration of my food plan was a basic lineup of three meals and an afternoon snack. I included foods I enjoy eating and are easy to prepare to make it as likely as possible that I would follow through on my choices at each meal. I also based most of my meals around whole foods that I know feel good in my body and create long-lasting energy. I minimized sugar, flour, and any other processed foods to limit the cravings and

hunger that result from blood sugar and insulin spikes. I learned from my coach that it is much easier to reign in eating when you have less desire and hunger for food. Choosing meals with whole foods and limiting refined foods was my plan for stabilizing hunger and cravings.

All these decisions were made by my conscious brain, well ahead of any eating. By making a food plan, I took spontaneous decisions around food out of the equation. The goal was to only eat what I had written down the night before. Any other suggestion to eat would be taken as an urge from my primitive brain. The plan itself was the first way I acted out my commitment to my future self. I prioritized thinking strategically about my long-term well-being instead of momentarily giving into cravings to eat.

Since I didn't want to make my food choices boring, I thought about ways to include delicious ingredients in moderation. Again, with planning, I decided on moderate portions of some indulgent foods throughout the week and practiced eating them with full attention. Part of this system involved limiting distractions while I ate so I could bring my full awareness to the pleasure in the food along with the pleasure in my body. I learned how much of certain foods—like chocolate or French fries—I could eat for pleasure without disrupting my body's well-being. Part of that well-being came from keeping urges for those foods to a minimum, so limiting the amounts I ate was vital.

In the absence of extra eating, the desire to eat would still sometimes bubble to the surface. When urges for food struck at the end of a stressful week or while I was out with a friend, I began considering my needs in that moment. If I wasn't hungry and my body felt light and energized, what was the desire there to tell me? I started wading through the undercurrent of my emotional life, making sense of how I felt and the ways food used to numb these emotions. I paid attention to desire and questioned how I could take care of myself without putting something else in my mouth.

Depending on the day, extra desire for food might point to a need to rest or relax. Lying down and closing my eyes worked wonders to give myself a break. In other instances, urges signaled my wanting to connect with loved ones, and I practiced listening and engaging more in conversation instead of always grabbing another bite. There were also times when it was important for me to get comfortable feeling boredom or disappointment without escaping them by eating. Staying connected to my body and becoming familiar with its emotional vibrations was a way to better learn the topography of my emotional landscape.

As I refined and tweaked this process for myself, I began teaching it to other food lovers inside my coaching business. One by one, I helped individuals craft their own plan and incorporate indulgences in a way that empowered them to feel in control.

After my first year in business, I recognized three basic shifts every food lover needs to make to balance eating for pleasure with maintaining pleasure in their bodies. I call these basics the three Cs of weight loss for food lovers. It's the trifecta of how to untangle the habit of overeating and regain empowerment around food and your body. These three basics are the foundation of what I teach all my new clients to change their relationship with food and themselves.

The First C: Commitment

You've already learned that commitment starts with a belief in yourself. But you might feel unsure about your ability to follow through on that belief. This is the time to act on your belief, so think about the word *discipline* as a substitute here for commitment. They are closely related when it comes to honoring a decision, goal, or objective you have for yourself. Many people who decide to work with me start with the assumption that they can't stay committed because they lack the discipline to see it through.

Take Simon, for instance, a former client of mine who is the CEO of a thriving aerospace company. Despite helping his company achieve tremendous growth and success and earning the title of CEO after years of professional striving, Simon described himself as a very undisciplined person.

"How can that be true," I asked him incredulously, "when you consider all your accomplishments?"

Simon thought for a moment. "No, you're right," he said decidedly. "I am very disciplined when it comes to getting what I want in business."

As we began working together, Simon discovered that eating was a kind of stress release. It was his way of decompressing, experiencing pleasure in the moment, and weaving in fun amid the intensity of work. During office hours, Simon's commitment to getting the job done was unwavering. After hours, he was all in on food.

Previous attempts to change his eating stemmed mainly from his desire to temporarily offset his weight gain. "If I'm honest," Simon confided on one call with me, "dieting ensures that I can eventually go back to eating again."

Using methods like 5:2 (in which you eat a balanced diet five days, then fast the other two) or Whole 30 (a plan of consistently eating a specific way for thirty days), Simon could intermittently lose weight for a period. There was no doubt from his success with these diets that he was able to commit temporarily.

Simon even suggested to me that these plans "worked" for him. He wondered whether he could work with me while still following one of those set diet formulas. It was not the first time I heard a client deem a previous diet successful.

My response to Simon was the same one I offer to everyone who comes to me needing help with weight loss, arguing that they have a plan that "works" for them. "If the plan works, why did you regain the weight?"

A way of eating is only as successful as your ability to continue doing it while still enjoying food and your life. Your relationship with food should naturally fit into your lifestyle, too, not something dependent on finding the "ideal time," right location, perfect foods, or otherwise stress-free situation. If your food plan doesn't mesh with real life, it's not going to truly work.

Remember, you first committed by deciding to believe you deserve more. You also have your compelling reasons why it matters to change your relationship with food. Acting on that decision and staying consistent with it will help you permanently change the habit of overeating and allow you to feel and look your best. Commitment itself is both a mindset as well as a set of actions. But it is not a perfect process. In fact, learning to stay committed happens when you embrace that failure is part of the process of learning.

If you believed it were possible to feel and look differently, would you be willing to try? Does at least a small part of you believe you deserve better than the life you're experiencing?

It's important to note here that the hundreds of people I've helped don't start out fully committed. If they already knew how to fully commit to themselves and follow through on different choices with food, they wouldn't need my help.

Instead, almost every person I talk to on a consultation asks almost the exact same question: "Do you think this could really work for someone like me?"

I get it. It's hard to go all in on something you've never been able to accomplish.

Think through your compelling reasons for wanting to change your relationship with food. By the way, no reason is unsuitable. If it's a reason you like and can stand behind, it's irrelevant if your reason is "I like the way I look five pounds lighter" or "I want to minimize the risk of diabetes." Your reason needs to matter to you, because it will form the backbone of your ability to exercise commitment. Remind yourself of that reason. Write it down. You don't need to justify your reason or explain it to anyone; just be sure *you* feel strongly about it.

Then, turn that commitment into a measurable goal. It can be a goal weight, or it might be fitting into a certain size of clothing. It could also be giving up snacking or desserts or making homemade meals instead of relying on fast food. Perhaps your goal is related to achieving more physical fitness, and eating has a direct impact on that. Pick one thing that will mark an external measure of your ability to be in control around food and feel good in your body. Make it a specific result that you achieve within a set time frame. The purpose of this goal is to give you something to aim for, even if you've never achieved it before.

When I discovered life coaching, I learned that we don't base our future success on what we've achieved in the past. Just because you haven't figured out yet how to be in your ideal body, feeling your best and empowered around food, doesn't mean it's not still possible. Your past is only an indication of what didn't work, not an indication of what you're capable of. To resolve your struggle with overeating once and for all, you need to be willing to try something new. Otherwise, you're just recreating the same results by resorting to past tactics.

Once a person steps into the realm of possibility, by believing "it might be possible for me," the brain opens to a new way of thinking. Instead of the old doubt of "I'll never be able to figure this out," or "Weight loss is the one area in which I can never succeed," what if the possibility still exists, and it's simply a matter of discovering it in a new way?

When you believe that "it might be possible for me," how does it make you feel? Notice that the emotion, whether it's hopeful, open, curious, excited, or something else, is much different than feeling defeated and resigned. Already this tiny seed of a thought opens up the possibility just by changing your emotional state—and then likely your actions.

The Second C: Consciousness

Now that you've decided on your goal, write down what you will eat each day to turn that commitment into a reality. This involves spending five minutes jotting down your breakfast, lunch, and dinner on a piece of paper. If you're not a breakfast eater, only write down the meals you typically eat in a day but make intentional choices around which foods and how much will nourish your body and be enjoyable to eat. Within the parameters of following your plan should be the basic principle of eating when you experience genuine hunger and stopping when you've satisfied that hunger. If you don't feel hungry, don't eat the lunch you planned until you do feel hungry. When you notice that subtle signal from your body that you've eaten just enough (before fullness), practice honoring that and stop, even if there is still food on your plate.

Mapping out your decisions in advance around what you will eat is a crucial step in developing awareness. Some of my clients will attempt to keep the idea of a plan in their head, without physically putting pen to paper. This usually comes from the common thought _I don't need to write it down._ But writing down the food you will eat accomplishes two things.

First, it begins to consciously manifest your commitment from a general idea in the brain to a physical statement of intent, thus making it more likely you will remember and beginning the momentum of following through.

Second, later it helps you clarify what you planned versus what you ate. Despite our general assumption that we will remember what we decided to eat, there are more than sixty thousand thoughts running through the brain at any given moment, and it's very likely you'll forget. A solid, written food plan keeps you conscious of your intention. It makes it obvious when you feel a spontaneous desire to override your best intentions. It sheds light on patterns of wanting to eat beyond physical nourishment.

The plan itself puts your conscious brain in charge, not as a rule enforcer but as a guide. Therefore, you should design a plan that's easy to commit to. Let go of ideas around what you think you *should* be eating, as well as any remnants of the old mentality suggesting "right" and "wrong" foods. An ideal food plan is one you can easily follow through on so you build trust in your ability to honor commitments to yourself. If it's unlikely you will eat salad with chicken for lunch, don't put it on your plan.

My clients run into trouble when they mistakenly think there is a "right" way to eat to get fast results. They think of their plan more as a set of rules, and this makes it less likely they will follow it in the moment. This is evident when they feel rebellious and think thoughts like *I don't want anyone telling me what to do*. But the sooner you let go of the false idea that there is a perfect plan, the easier it will be to become more conscious in your eating.

To do it right or perfectly, or to adhere to some old notion of what a food plan should look like, many people by default will create an unrealistic food plan in the beginning. No wonder they feel resistant to doing any of the things they decided! The plan backfires when, after feeling deprived and rebellious, these people overeat all the food they restricted themselves from planning.

I make sure my clients understand that nothing has gone wrong when this happens. It's a natural response to decades of learning how to white-knuckle your way through a diet that omits most of the food you love. Feeling rebellious toward a plan you created for yourself is a useful clue of how you're thinking about food, and it brings to the surface the first of many old beliefs that probably don't serve you and the relationship you want most with food.

This is one initial example of how the food plan helps develop consciousness. Your response to your own plan helps reveal your current thinking and show you what you're believing. When the decisions around food are made in advance, it reduces the mental chatter about what to eat. Still, urges for unplanned food will happen. This stirring of desire is an important part of the experience. When you pay attention to that wanting, instead of reacting to it by eating, it's a conscious experience of being present with your emotions.

Those urges are the emotion of desire. For many people, desire feels like a fast restlessness, almost an antsy sensation coursing through the body. The unconscious habit might be to grab something to eat to quell this feeling, to get rid of it and take the edge off. But when your daily plan doesn't include the food you're craving that minute, it's a beautiful opportunity to process feelings naturally instead.

Staying conscious looks like first noticing the emotional vibration in your body of desire, or even just the suggestion from your brain of *I want something to eat*. Many people who struggle with overeating are so well practiced at just eating out of habit when they feel that way, not questioning whether they are even hungry, that noticing the thought or feeling in the moment is challenging at first. This is how the plan is a useful tool for creating awareness.

When food is off the table (i.e., not on the plan), what's left is just you and your feelings.

Paying attention to urges helps you discover the pattern in your need to eat when you're not hungry. It can help you investigate the void that food is filling and explore what's there. What do you truly need and desire in that moment?

Experiences of overeating can be opportunities instead of problems when you're willing to bring conscious awareness back into the equation. I remind my clients that this, too, is part of staying committed to the process of change. Commitment and consciousness are not just reserved for when all is well and you're following through on your plan. It's just as important to employ these two things when your plan goes awry. In fact, it can be one of the most powerful parts of your learning.

The way to stay conscious after overeating is by first being willing to accept what happened. There is no changing the past or undoing your choice to eat. We know that regret doesn't lead you anywhere good, so practice just acknowledging that you made the choice to eat and can now turn it into a useful experience.

There are three key questions to ask yourself to bring consciousness back to your choices around food. It's best to go through this exercise of self-reflection within the same day of overeating to give you the best chance of recalling all the details.

1. What led up to you deciding to overeat?
Take a moment to think about what was happening earlier in the day before you put food in your mouth. Was there a stressful experience at work or with a family member? Were you around delicious food, or did you watch someone else eat something you wanted? How were you feeling right before you decided to eat? What thoughts convinced you to turn to food? Consider whether this time of day, when you decided to overeat, is part of a regular pattern of overeating.

2. What exactly did you eat?

Your brain quickly wants to take an experience of overeating and move it into the unconscious, where it can be stored as a habit worth repeating again for that dopamine hit. In answer to this question, you might be tempted to answer in a general way with something like "I had some cookies." But it's important that you be as specific as possible in listing every piece of food you consumed, sequentially, including any little bites or tastes. The objective is to bring the act of mindless eating to the forefront of your brain where you can consciously observe and notice what happened.

Pay attention to any thoughts that led you to keep eating and also to the thinking that finally stopped you from putting food in your mouth. Consider what the experience of tasting the food was like and how pleasurable it felt. Perhaps your brain suggested at first that you would just have "one little bite," and it turned out to be four cookies, two mini peanut butter cups, one handful of cashews, one glass of wine, and two bites of a blueberry muffin. Reflect on whether choosing to eat the food helped you resolve or not resolve your feelings in the moment. What was the overall experience like, even after you finished eating? Bring awareness to the truth of what giving into that craving for food creates both during the eating and the hours that follow it.

3. What are some useful insights from exploring this incident of mindless eating that you can apply to future situations?

The second C of weight loss also pertains to elevating the level of consciousness when eating meals on your plan. Desire and eating are so tightly intertwined that if you're not fully paying attention, you can slip into mindlessness when eating food that tastes especially good or that you're particularly hungry for. You'll notice this happening when you start eating fast, your fork rushing to scoop up bites before your mouth has finished chewing.

Gobbling your food is a reaction to desire, even when the food is something you intentionally decided to have. It's a natural reaction your brain has when you're hungry, see delicious food, and make the connection that it's time to eat. I notice this happening while I'm standing in the kitchen, beginning to prepare my food. If I'm not careful, I may even serve myself a larger portion than I need because I'm reacting to the restless feeling of wanting to eat.

This is when you also might feel tempted to nibble before sitting down for your actual meal. All the neural synapses are firing, telling you it's time to eat, and the restless energy building in your body can make it seem like an emergency that can't wait.

When you notice that quickening, it's the perfect time to actively calm yourself down and regain conscious awareness before putting food in your mouth. I do this by reconnecting to my breathing and slowing it down through deep, slow inhales and exhales. I gently remind myself that there is no rush, and I put my fork down while I pause and set the intention to thoroughly enjoy my first bite of food.

Conscious eating serves two important roles in stopping the habit of eating too much. The first is that it helps you taste more of the flavor of your food when you're focusing on all the senses and bringing heightened attention to the experience of eating.

This makes it completely worth it if you're someone who loves food as much as I do. To have more pleasure from what you're putting into your mouth, you need to be more conscious of how it tastes. Shoveling mouthfuls of food from a place of urgent desire misses the opportunity to taste and delight in each morsel, bite by bite.

I remind myself of this when I feel like I'm in a rush to gobble up my meal. I'm missing out on the experience of pleasure if I don't slow down and savor what's in front of me. When you taste your food fully, it goes a long way in helping you feel satisfied sooner. This is the second role conscious eating plays in helping you lose weight. Not only do you feel satisfied with the experience of tasting your food by slowly eating and savoring it, but you also give your body the chance to catch up with digestion. You're more likely to notice the satiety cues your body sends when you've had enough.

I give my clients some prompts to use to guide themselves through the act of conscious eating. There are some simple questions you, too, can use to talk yourself through slowing down and eating with awareness.

Sample Questions for Conscious Eating

1. What am I noticing about this first bite of food in terms of appearance, smell, taste, feel, and even the way it sounds while I eat it?
2. Do I enjoy the way this food tastes?
3. Do I want to keep eating this food?
4. What do I notice about the flavor of this food after the first few bites?

> 5. How is my body feeling after I am halfway through eating this portion of food?
> 6. Have I had enough of this food, or do I need more?

Each step (or bite) of the way is a chance to reconsider your choice to keep eating. If the food doesn't taste good, give yourself permission not to eat it. When your body signals in its subtle way that it's content and satisfied, practice concluding the eating experience even if there is still emotional hunger (desire) for more to eat. This is how you start teaching yourself to be satisfied with less food without sacrificing the pleasure in eating.

Learning the art of conscious eating helps undo the notion that more food is better, or that feeling physically stuffed equates with satisfaction. It keeps you attuned to your body and the amount of nourishment it needs for your ideal size. Conscious eating allows you to indulge in the food you love, fully delight in it, and learn how to moderate your appetite based on physical cues. Once you develop the habit of eating food slowly, mindfully, and in proportion to what feels like just enough in your body, you unlearn the idea that you need bigger portions, multiple refills, or extra courses at a restaurant to reach a point you can feel satisfied with.

The Third C: Consistency

Each of the three Cs is a necessary key in unlocking your ability to reach your ideal size enjoyably and sustainably. I created these keys by realizing the major obstacles that prevent mainstream diets from working. Most of us don't struggle with finding an eating plan, or even losing weight, if it's just for a few days.

When clients come to me for one-on-one support, it's because they can't figure out how to do all of it *consistently*. They are not used to prioritizing themselves and knowing how to commit to making their goals a reality. Dieting has taught them how to eat a particular way that feels more like white-knuckling instead of a satisfying eating experience. Using willpower to tough it out through a quick-fix diet leaves many of us crashing and burning once we no longer have the stamina to fend off deprivation. It sets us up to fail and inevitably revert to overeating.

Again, if a way of eating is not something you can easily follow day after day, it's not a viable plan for weight loss. The sticking point here is that a food plan works only insofar as you're capable of staying consistent with it. We are used to believing that diets are short-term strategies, but to both lose and maintain a lower weight, you need to eat in a way that maintains that new size.

The first time I realized this, I panicked. I imagined being on a restricted diet for the rest of my life, without the joy of indulging in delicious food. It felt like someone was taking away my childhood blanket—the one I carried around daily for comfort and hugged tightly until its yarn pulled apart and frayed at the seams. No one wants to feel like they've been handed a life sentence of following a bland, boring diet in the name of being thin.

I certainly didn't.

I've shared on my podcast a certainty that I still stand behind. If given the choice between being thin or delighting in the food I love, the decision is unanimous. Food wins every time.

But what if it doesn't need to be an either/or decision? This is where consistency comes in.

Inherent in the struggle most people have with staying consistent on a diet is the underlying assumption that weight loss needs to involve a restrictive, limited food plan. In coaching sessions with my clients, we spend ample time unlearning old ideas about what "works" to lose weight and focus instead on how to create something we can stay consistent with.

Consistency is vital to long-term success, but it flies in the face of what people generally want to believe about weight loss. We want to take temporary action, in short bursts, and see dramatic results quickly. No wonder this leads to drastic measures like overexercising to burn calories, or undereating at one meal to "save up" for overeating later on. Old-school diets promote a disordered approach to eating that is almost impossible to stay consistent with if your goal is to create a relationship with food that makes you feel and look good.

Consistency matters because no plan truly works permanently if you can only do it for a brief period. Equally important is the role consistency plays in establishing the internal habits that create empowerment and freedom around food. The more regularly you think intentionally, process emotions naturally, and continue taking action even when it's uncomfortable, the more ingrained the new relationship with food becomes.

Food for Thought

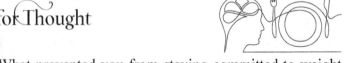

1. What prevented you from staying committed to weight loss in the past?
2. What stops you from feeling ready to change your relationship with food now?

3. If you believe that setbacks were part of the learning process, what would you be willing to try?
4. What is one simple change you can make today that might help you be more conscious about what you eat?
5. What's the risk of deciding to put off making this change?
6. How might your life be different if you finally experience freedom from food?

Chapter 6:

Roadblocks to Freedom from Food

Most diets teach us only what we need to know to lose weight. What's missing, and what we usually struggle with, is how to make the results permanent. Commitment, consciousness, and consistency make up the practice of trying, failing, and learning from setbacks. We always have the primitive brain coming along for the ride, and finding our way back to the three Cs looks more like a crooked path and never like a perfectly straight journey. What I've learned is that there are common obstacles most food lovers face when it comes to staying consistent in this process. Understanding these diversions on your own path may make it easier to sidestep them as often as they arise.

Food Obsession

The habit of overeating stems from an emphasis on food and eating as a way to heighten pleasure, distract yourself, or just make yourself feel better. Food momentarily fills the void, but it's never deeply satisfying, so it leads to a larger emotional appetite. Traditional diets encourage an obsession with food and seeking something outside yourself to create wellness. Scouring meal plans that promote the right combination of food or swear off certain food groups entirely leads you to believe that it's just a matter of eating the right way. Tracking calories, macros, points, or carbs also leads to an overemphasis on food.

I remember the old days of dieting when I thought drinking a SlimFast shake for breakfast and lunch was the magic bullet for success. I religiously stocked up on my favorite chocolate flavor—which, compared to the chicken and broccoli dinner I obediently ate every night, tasted like a treat.

Back then, I believed that as long as I had my shake and chicken dinner, I was safe. But I fantasized about the day when I'd be able to eat some pancakes for breakfast or pizza for dinner. Those foods were forbidden according to the way I understood the diet, and my yearning to eat them only grew bigger.

I was tethered to my two-shake-a-day plan, and that structure provided a false sense of security. It relied on my ability to resist and avoid all other noncompliant foods to succeed. In the beginning, when I was highly motivated to lose weight, it was easy to stick with it because I was so frustrated with feeling terrible. But I never learned how to include food I loved, and the mental chatter around all the delicious foods I missed was relentless.

When I dieted, I was either obsessing about the food I was allowed to eat for weight loss or fantasizing about all the food that was forbidden. Most of my thinking was still about food, instead of being curious about my body. I still thought the solution had to do with food instead of realizing my body had the answers. This obsession was time-consuming, and it ultimately led back to overeating every time.

Willpower

So many people I speak with still believe that willpower is necessary to weight loss. They are unwilling to even try something different because they believe they aren't disciplined enough to make it work. To clarify, willpower and commitment are not the same thing. Remember, commitment begins with a belief in yourself, and then a willingness to act on behalf of that belief with consistency. Commitment to yourself involves failing at times, knowing it will not be a perfect process, learning from setbacks, and continuing on with the journey.

Commitment allows you to slowly untangle the habit, while willpower is using sheer force to just get through the tough parts. Willpower relies on resisting your emotions, avoiding food, and gritting your teeth until you reach the finish line. It's a tense, exhausting experience. On the other hand, commitment involves meeting yourself at every step along the way, accepting the signals from your body, and treating yourself with kindness as you understand what you need.

I was a competitive swimmer for many years, and I always thought of myself as a disciplined person. One might argue that I have more willpower than most. I don't know how you measure it, but I think I'm especially good at enduring challenges.

So why, then, did I always run out of stamina when it came to dieting?

When people rely on willpower for weight loss, it's a way of pushing through something hard to get it over with. According to *Britannica Dictionary*, *willpower* is defined as "strong determination that allows you to do something difficult." Conjuring up that determination always made my experience of dieting feel like a big struggle. Enduring another day of bland eating, eating less in hopes the scale would budge, and fighting off thoughts about sweets all cost a lot of energy. And if I was able to get through the gauntlet of dieting this way, I inevitably wanted to reward myself with an abundance of all my favorite foods.

Using willpower was exhausting, and it robbed me of an opportunity to understand my body and enjoy the process of helping it feel good. When my energy was depleted from trying to power my way through eating perfectly, it wasn't available to manage cravings when they did pop up. Willpower ultimately increased my desire to come running back to all my favorite foods, instead of giving me any real sense of authority over food and my body.

The antidote was so simple, so organic, that it's surprising it took me so long to discover it: My body has the answers I need, and I just need to listen to it. Food, calories, points, shakes, macros, and all the other external forces do not need to be controlled when I am noticing what my body is telling me. Through its hardwired programming, my body already knows what it needs to feel its best. Releasing the pressure that comes from willpower also allows the body to relax. It makes it much easier to shed extra physical weight when the mental weight comes off first.

Negative Self-Talk

If obsessing about food and white-knuckling my way through a diet didn't make the experience miserable enough, my own self-criticism topped it off. I chastised myself for eating too much after a hard day, felt guilty when I couldn't follow the plan flawlessly, and was ashamed that I still struggled with weight loss.

I didn't realize that engaging with my inner critic was optional—that it was a common thought pattern, and I could choose to disengage instead of agreeing with negativity about myself. When I started working with my coach, she said to me, "Why are you allowing yourself to speak to yourself that way?"

Until then, I never knew I had a choice and could shut down the incessant voice of judgment.

Self-criticism pretends to keep us in line and on track, but instead it erodes our sense of self. For many people, it is such an ingrained habit that it's accepted as the truth, instead of questioned or dismissed altogether. Instead of creating a sense of trust, it does the opposite and creates a relationship that is anything but enjoyable.

When I used to verbally beat myself up, it made me less likely to want to care for myself. It mentally weighed me down and had me running back to food to escape myself. The more I internally punished myself and believed I wasn't measuring up, the more I devalued my own self-worth.

Negative self-talk adds a layer of misery to a process that should be about self-care and nurturing the body. It wears down the spirit and adds an unnecessary load of mental baggage. When I learned how easy it was to let go of, I instantly felt lighter.

Through my own inner script, I practiced talking back to myself. If my primitive brain hissed, "You shouldn't have done that," I would respond right away with "That's not useful."

When my inner critic taunted and said, "You'll never be able to figure this out," I retorted, "We don't speak to ourselves that way."

As I slowly changed the narrative of my own dialogue, something miraculous happened. My inner critic piped down and gave up on its rants. When I stopped engaging and spiraling downward into a pit of self-loathing, the negative self-talk was no longer effective at leading me back to overeating.

Now, the voice of self-judgment rarely surfaces. When it does, the first little squeak of criticism is snuffed out by my voice of reason.

Since you now understand the obstacles, let's next discuss the key steps to arriving at freedom around food.

The Trifecta of Food Freedom

The more you take the focus off food as the problem and the solution, the closer you get to experiencing freedom. This happens naturally when you get used to recreating pleasure in your body at every meal. Knowing how it feels to be light, energized, and nourished and how you recreate that by your eating is the secret sauce.

There are three things that enable freedom from food to take hold and dissolve the shackles of overeating.

1. End the obsession around food and put the focus on your body.
Your brain might still offer suggestions of what you should eat. Something sweet after dinner, another slice of pizza, or some cheese and crackers during a break could pop up as sentences in

your head. But until you start engaging with these thoughts, they have no control over what you choose to eat next.

Freedom comes from letting these thoughts go, like passing ships sailing down the current of your mind. Spontaneous thoughts about eating, unrelated to physical hunger, are the voice of your emotional appetite. By releasing the tantalizing feed of thoughts when you're not hungry, you get back to the peace and quiet of your body.

Beware of obsession around so-called "healthy" foods, too. Micromanaging your plate to get faster results, or to feel virtuous, is a losing battle since it keeps you overthinking food instead of how you feel. Take notes on how certain foods make you feel, and whether any of them disrupt the sense of calm and peace of well-being. Notice whether foods, usually with processed ingredients, increase your natural hunger or elevate cravings. Choosing too many of those foods may offset the pleasure you want to experience and the sense of ease that comes with less thinking about food.

2. Let go of any fear around hunger.

Like food obsession, this skill can be a process of unlearning old ways of thinking. Fear around hunger is an instinctive response many of us have for good reason. The primitive brain interprets hunger as a danger to our survival, so we are not programmed to feel comfortable around it. Couple that hardwiring with societal beliefs that prolonged hunger effects metabolism, and it's no surprise that we panic at the first grumble or growl.

It's normal for many people to feel a sense of urgency around hunger, as if it's an emergency that needs immediate resolving. The problem with making food choices from a place of urgency is that it leads to mindlessness, fast eating, and being disconnected from the physical cues of your body. It also perpetuates the idea that hunger is a problem that needs to be solved immediately.

You can retrain your response to hunger with a little mindset work, and dropping fear and urgency allows you to have ease and control around food and your body. For instance, you can detach your thinking about hunger from the actual physical experience of it in your body. Like a type of meditation, you observe the sensation of growling or gnawing in your stomach without engaging in the thought that it's a problem to feel that way.

The more comfortable you get with noticing hunger by itself, the easier it is to see that it comes in waves and never escalates into an intense matter or life or death. When prolonged, hunger pangs usually diminish, then evolve into lack of energy or an inability to focus. Note: The point of understanding hunger is never to ride it out and underfeed yourself, but rather to get comfortable with what it feels like and how you can experience it without overeating.

Feeling in control and at peace with hunger releases another layer of tension in your relationship with food. It strengthens your connection to your body because you more easily identify what it needs and how to best care for it.

3. Soften resistance to emotions.
Just like hunger, emotions have a physical manifestation in your body. A vibration of energy occurs when you feel some-

thing like sadness, anger, excitement, or curiosity. Some emotions feel more uncomfortable than others, mainly because you probably don't have enough practice experiencing them. Many of us were not taught that it's okay to express our feelings, or how to notice them in the body so they can process naturally. Instead, many of us were taught to avoid or distract ourselves from our feelings.

Eating is one of the most typical ways to do this, because it's easy, convenient, and socially acceptable. When you're not familiar with what it's like to feel sad, and you've never observed the sensation of it detached from your thinking about it, it can seem unsafe. Your primitive brain recognizes unfamiliar feelings as dangerous and scary and out of instinct will create resistance to them. Out of resistance, you may also feel the urgency to eat to relax and feel better.

Eating to avoid unfamiliar feelings perpetuates the cycle of escaping yourself and neglecting your body. Overfeeding yourself to take the edge off the discomfort of an emotional vibration only adds an extra layer of discomfort on top of the discomfort of your feelings. It also ingrains the habit that certain feelings need to be avoided with food and increases the desire to eat when you're not physically hungry.

When you eat to avoid feelings, it doesn't provide the emotional or physical relief you want. But by learning to observe emotions and how they take shape in your body, in the same meditative way I mentioned with hunger, you gain competency and confidence in managing the full spectrum of feelings. The benefits are twofold, since you not only understand yourself better by listening to your feelings, but you also give those emotions the space to process naturally through you. The result is a lightness of being and peace of mind.

The trifecta of freedom around food is what helps you ultimately let go of physical and mental weight so the journey of getting back to your ideal body is one of ease and peace. Resolving the mental struggle with food is what allows the physical struggle with your body to resolve and take care of it itself.

Learning the reasons why you turn to food when your body doesn't need it is a journey of self-awareness. Overeating distracts us from our deepest needs since food pretends to be an easy solution when we want to feel better. We're used to believing that the problem is either food or the weight gain itself, but those two things only disguise the deeper issue. When my clients begin this work, they still believe, based on an old diet mentality, that weight loss will be a process of micromanaging their body. It's not until they do the emotional work of understanding the void that food fills that they realize the heart of this work is about rediscovering themselves.

Identifying your *emotional appetite* is an important step in deciding the type of relationship you want to have with food. Maybe your current relationship with food is the one you want, but how do you know?

You know by the way it makes you feel and by being in touch with your body. Your body is your anchor, grounding you in the reality of how you feel physically and emotionally. It will tell you the truth of your life experience based on your emotional and physical wellness.

In Part Two, we investigate the spectrum of the emotional appetite. Through the stories of some of my past clients, we look at the common reasons food lovers turn to food for emotional reasons. Together, we decode what is driving you to eat and decipher the needs you have below the surface of the habit. Step-by-step, I guide you through the process I use to recognize the habit of overeating, unravel it, and get back in touch with your body.

Food for Thought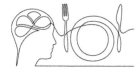

1. What has been your experience of using willpower around food?
2. In what situations do you engage in negative self-talk?
3. If you knew that failing along the way was part of the process, how might you respond differently to yourself?
4. If you believed that you could figure out how to feel better and be more in control around food, how would you make sense of an experience of overeating?
5. What is one example of an emotion you tend to escape by eating?
6. What is some existing evidence that you know how to stop eating and be connected to your body?
7. What's one step you can take today to being more focused on your body and less on food?

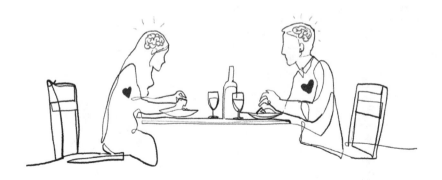

Part II:

Decoding Your Emotional Appetite

Chapter 7:

The Four Emotional Appetites

When Karen started working with me, she had no idea how to eat to be in her ideal body. Her go-to menu was eating what she called "kids' food," and boiled down to whatever her teenage sons and her husband were in the mood for. As a child, Karen was always identified as the "big" kid when compared to her two brothers. She grew up with a mom who relied mainly on fast food for meals, and she taught Karen by example how to zone out by eating. Karen ate what was available, and she ate to join in on the eating. It's what she knew.

When she came to me, she had spent years believing she would always be in what she described as a "big body." That belief was reinforced by her parents, who described her size as "just part of the family genetics." Yet it didn't feel right to Karen. The older she got, the worse her body felt—not just physically, but also emotionally. It's no surprise that when Karen felt physically unwell, it was hard for her to emotionally feel well.

As she started the process of uncovering her love language with food, Karen began to make sense of the role food usually played in her life. Instead of feeling frustrated or ashamed about her body, she began to understand it. She learned how to honor it by listening below the surface when food was no longer taking up all the space.

Karen easily began losing weight, too. Initially, it surprised her how easily she could lose several pounds a week because it was a different experience than the usual diet she often resorted to. She practiced focusing on her body instead of on food, and at first it felt foreign to do so.

"I feel like I'm learning a new language," she told me about four weeks into our time together.

Food was indeed her primary love language, and in my experience, this language has multiple dialects. Specifically, clients tend to use food to meet one of four types of emotional appetites: security, escape, connection, and pleasure.

- The emotional appetite of *security* says, "Food will make me feel safe."
- The emotional appetite of *escape* says, "I deserve a treat."
- The emotional appetite of *connection* says, "I might stand out if I don't join in."
- The emotional appetite of *pleasure* says, "More is better."

In the next several chapters, I cover some specific types of emotional needs and how others have successfully disentangled their emotional appetite from food.

Food for Thought

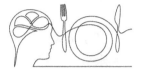

Which of the emotional appetites listed above sound familiar to you? To find out, I invite you to take the quiz below.

Quiz: Emotional Appetite Tendency Score (EATS)
The following quiz is designed to help you gain self-awareness of your emotional appetite. There are no right or wrong answers, and your relationship with food will continue to evolve over time. Respond to the following sixteen statements from the perspective of how much you currently relate to/identify with each one.

Circle the best response for each statement from 0 to 4.

1. When I go to a party, I spend much of the time huddled with friends near the food/drinks.
0 = Never 1 = Rarely 2 = Occasionally 3 = Usually 4 = Always

2. After a long or challenging day, I make a beeline to the kitchen or a restaurant.
0 = Never 1 = Rarely 2 = Occasionally 3 = Usually 4 = Always

3. I keep snacks/treats stored in a special place.
0 = Never 1 = Rarely 2 = Occasionally 3 = Usually 4 = Always

4. I am already scheduling the next great meal.
0 = Never 1 = Rarely 2 = Occasionally 3 = Usually 4 = Always

5. I finish what is on my plate because it would be a waste not to.
0 = Never 1 = Rarely 2 = Occasionally 3 = Usually 4 = Always

6. I order/prepare extra because it might be needed.
0 = Never 1 = Rarely 2 = Occasionally 3 = Usually 4 = Always

7. When I get bad news or am upset, a little of my favorite food can help take the edge off.
0 = Never 1 = Rarely 2 = Occasionally 3 = Usually 4 = Always

8. Meeting with a friend/family seems boring if food is not involved.
0 = Never 1 = Rarely 2 = Occasionally 3 = Usually 4 = Always

9. Something sweet is a perfect way to end a meal.
0 = Never 1 = Rarely 2 = Occasionally 3 = Usually 4 = Always

10. There are certain dishes I love to eat as they remind me of my mom/dad/(other).
0 = Never 1 = Rarely 2 = Occasionally 3 = Usually 4 = Always

11. Most events I attend involve eating and drinking.
0 = Never 1 = Rarely 2 = Occasionally 3 = Usually 4 = Always

12. I work hard and deserve a treat and a little "me time" with a favorite food.
0 = Never 1 = Rarely 2 = Occasionally 3 = Usually 4 = Always

13. After completing a project/event, food can serve as a good reward.

0 = Never 1 = Rarely 2 = Occasionally 3 = Usually 4 = Always

14. I might stand out or offend someone if I don't join in eating/drinking when others are.

0 = Never 1 = Rarely 2 = Occasionally 3 = Usually 4 = Always

15. There are some foods that I see or smell and just need to have it all.

0 = Never 1 = Rarely 2 = Occasionally 3 = Usually 4 = Always

16. I find myself searching the kitchen to find the perfect bite to satisfy a craving.

0 = Never 1 = Rarely 2 = Occasionally 3 = Usually 4 = Always

Now add up your responses for the questions noted in the respective parentheses and put the total next to each emotional appetite type:

Security (3, 5, 6, 10) = _____

Escape (2, 7, 12, 13) = _____

Connection (1, 8, 11, 14) = _____

Pleasure (4, 9, 15, 16) = _____

The larger your number in a certain emotional appetite area, the higher your Emotional Appetite Tendency Score (EATS) is in that area. Again, there is no "correct" number or score distribution. As you work to change your relationship with food, you might enjoy taking this quiz again to see if you have decreased your tendency in any areas.

as of what she should be able to eat for her size and the kind diet it takes to lose weight.

That old way of thinking was not getting those last ten ounds off. After struggling for several years to lose the same en pounds, Maureen was close to giving up on herself. She asked me if maybe at her age (mid-sixties), it was unrealistic to think she could get to her ideal weight. It wasn't the first time I heard of someone struggling for so long to lose the last few pounds. It occurs when entitled thinking around food is at its peak. The superficial attempts at dieting and focusing solely on external cues cease to work, and many people give up.

One of the telltale signs with Maureen was that she rarely felt hungry. My first assumption was that she was eating too much. When I recommended that she write down a food plan and keep track of what she ate, Maureen flatly responded, "I don't need to do that; I eat more or less the same thing every day." Maureen believed that having a general idea in her head of what she ate was enough to lose weight.

Defiance against planning wasn't the only obstacle for her. Questioning the amount of food she was consuming also made Maureen feel defensive. "I only eat healthy foods—and very modest portions," she fired back at me.

Maureen was deeply attached to not only her familiar way of eating, but also her well-established beliefs about what she should be allowed to eat. During our coaching together, we dug deeper into why she felt unwilling to change her approach to eating. "Food has always been a source of security for me," she confided, "and it reminds me of my mother." Maureen recounted her experience as a college student living

Chapter 8:

Security

Maureen came to me wanting to lose those l[...] ten pounds. She had a petite frame, and [...] a child she had been naturally slender. Wit[h] age, she found it harder to eat whatever she felt like without gaining weight. During the COVID-19 pandemic she turned to food for comfort and easily gained fifteen pounds. No matter what she tried, five pounds was the most she could lose, and then the scale stopped moving. That extra weight kept Maureen feeling disconnected from herself and dissatisfied with her life.

The process of embodying her authentic self required Maureen to pay more attention to her body and less attention to food. It meant dialing in her precise level of satiety instead of relying on visual portion sizes as her guide. For someone who was not eating large quantities of food to begin with, this brought up a certain type of resistance. Maureen was used to preconceived in Boston and spending evenings at a local Greek restaurant run by an elderly couple. "The owner would come to my table and sit with me, and his wife made green beans that were identical to my mother's." Spending time at the restaurant eased her feelings of homesickness and made Maureen feel more secure.

When the pandemic hit, Maureen's first instinct was to stock up on her favorite food. "I knew if I had the ingredients I needed, everything would be fine," she said assuredly. "Food was my sense of safety when everything else felt uncertain."

Food connected Maureen to her mother, and she felt protected and loved when she thought about the foods she grew up with. Maureen was comforted by the taste of those familiar foods or the smell of ingredients that reminded her of being at home in the kitchen with her mom. She carried that memory—and the belief that food created security—into adulthood.

During the pandemic, baking her mother's recipe for challah every Friday evening gave Maureen a cozy feeling of being wrapped in a warm blanket. Since she was isolated from friends and family, eating was a way she felt connected and safe during a time when fear over getting sick preoccupied her thinking. When life returned to normal, Maureen was fifteen pounds heavier and frustrated that it didn't easily come off.

Letting go of certain foods felt very challenging for Maureen. She looked forward to the two almond cookies and milk tea she enjoyed in the middle of the day, which was a ritual she used to share with her mother. Maureen found it hard to believe that giving up the two quarter-size sweets would really make a difference in her weight.

Maureen, like many people I work with, felt entitled to food. Many of us have ingrained ideas about what kinds of food, and how much, we should be able to eat and still have the body we desire. Preconceptions around "good" and "bad" foods, standard caloric intake, and what constitutes an ideal portion size keep many people focused on external indicators of what works for weight loss. Yet all these socially accepted standards ignore the individual experience of someone in their unique body.

Instead of focusing on what our bodies say is enough, and what foods feel nourishing when we eat them, we end up basing our choices around old metrics. It's normal for us to resist the idea that what we are eating may be too much for our body. That suggestion often triggers a scarcity response in the brain—the feeling that we might not have enough food or will feel deprived if we give up any bites. The primal response of fear around not having enough is part of our hardwired survival thinking, and it's an opportunity to acknowledge that nothing has gone wrong when the brain offers this.

But in every instance when I've encouraged a client to challenge their familiar way of eating, they are surprised by the true experience of stepping into that fear. With Maureen, for instance, I broached the change in a very delicate way. Knowing there is a tendency to resist what's comfortable, and a fear of not having enough food, I encouraged her to step into the fear of trying something new with baby steps.

Core Belief: *Food will make me feel safe.*

When Maureen turned to food for security, it came from the common belief that "food will make me feel better." This universal assumption takes many different forms when it comes to motivating us to overeat. In Maureen's example, it was tied to her sense of safety and security.

Key Mindset Shift: *I can support myself.*

This core belief made it hard for Maureen to let go of some of her eating, but we bridged the discomfort by thinking of it as an experiment so she didn't think she was giving up her beloved food permanently. I had her practice thinking, *This is plenty*, when she served herself a bit less at meals, and it shifted her focus toward really enjoying the planned amount on her plate. It helped her eat slowly and savor the food, knowing that portion was what she had to enjoy. By slowing down, she could more easily hear her body's response when the gently nudge of satiety happened.

Key Emotional Shift: From Entitled to Compassionate

To wade into the fear around less food, and the feelings of insecurity that came with it, it was important to not make a huge leap. Part of this process was helping Maureen create a sense of safety within herself and learn to trust her body. To do that, she needed to start small, in a way that felt doable at first. By approaching one meal at a time and lessening the food by a fraction, Maureen could explore the difference in her body with more ease. Knowing she could eat a little more if she felt hungry again after an hour further helped her to be willing to test out this new way of eating. Instead of feeling entitled to a set amount of food, Maureen became curious about how her body would respond to a new amount. When she felt curious, she explored the unfamiliar territory of a new satiety point and the difference in how her body felt.

The Process

1. Decide to experiment with one meal and make the commitment to yourself the day before. Write down what you will eat and have an idea in your mind of the typical portion to serve yourself. Write down next to your plan, "I will serve myself two spoonfuls less."

2. At the time of your meal, as you're serving your food, remind yourself that "you need less than you think." There can be a tendency when your brain sees the food in front of you to experience an urge to dish up a bit more ahead of time. Knowing you want to connect with your body first before deciding how much food you need, anticipate that the urge will be there so you don't mindlessly revert back to the old habit.

3. Before taking your first bite, set your intention to savor and slowly eat by pausing and reminding yourself, "This is plenty." If you notice any fear bubble up, gently remind yourself, "If I'm hungry in another hour, I will just eat a little more."

4. Notice what happens to your hunger as you eat and be curious about when you reach a satiety point before fullness. With less food, the hunger may be satisfied and replaced with a new lightness that might seem unfamiliar at first.

5. An hour after completing your meal, be curious about whether the hunger returns. Connect with your body and check for any signs of physical hunger to see whether you need to eat a bit more.

In Maureen's case, experimenting with an unfamiliar way of eating yielded incredible results. Like many of my clients who try this, she noticed that an hour later she wasn't hungry at all. She felt slightly more hunger four hours later, before her next meal, which made it more satisfying to sit down and nourish her body. Prior to this experiment, Maureen rarely felt much hunger at all. This, too, was a clue that she had been eating a little more than her body needed to be ten pounds lighter.

Experiencing a touch more hunger was a positive sign that Maureen's body could be encouraged to start burning fat again for energy. She also loved the sensation of feeling lighter overall in her body. She noticed that when she wasn't full or overfed, she had more energy and also slept better at night. The safer Maureen felt eating a little less and still being satisfied, the more willing she was to incorporate this approach into every meal she ate.

The compound effect of eating two bites less at every meal was dramatic. Maureen quickly dropped two pounds within the first week. Knowing she had figured out the solution to getting the last ten pounds off, she was even more motivated than before. She developed confidence in her ability to connect with her body and honor how she felt. She created security and safety within herself, which empowered her in a way she had never experienced before around food.

In six weeks, she released the ten pounds and told me, "I feel more like myself these days than I have in a long time."

Food for Thought

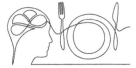

Do your own experiment to challenge your familiar assumptions around food and what you feel entitled to.

1. Choose one meal, and either change the quantity of how much you eat or the kind of food you're consuming. If you're trying to get closer to your ideal body weight, be willing to question what feels good in your body.
2. After eating a bit less, or trying some new kinds of food, observe like a scientist the results of this test. What's different about how your body feels right after finishing the last bite of food?
3. How would you describe your satiety?
4. What do you notice an hour later about your satisfaction level?

Chapter 9:

Escape

Tom identified himself as an overachiever. He ran a successful IT company, was married, and was the father of two young boys. Beginning in graduate school, Tom set his sights on landing a prestigious job and working his way up the ranks. Food was always a passion of his, and his free time was spent exploring some of the best restaurants in Manhattan. At 6 foot 2 inches, Tom's healthy appetite for eating never posed a problem—until he was under stress.

During a consultation with Tom, I learned that his relationship with food ebbed and flowed depending on his workload. Overeating was his favorite coping mechanism to handle an ambitious agenda for his company and juggling the responsibilities of coaching sports for his kids. Eating was a way to "get through" an overly scheduled calendar that left no downtime for Tom to enjoy the fruits of his labor. Because food was a natural love of his, he thought of overeating as "me time," or the chance to get away, albeit briefly, from the stressors of a packed life. Without the time and space to relax, unwind, and consider how he felt, Tom mindlessly turned to the pantry for relief.

Eventually the results of eating too much forced Tom to pay attention. Often gaining upwards of sixty pounds above his ideal weight, Tom had to face the reality of how escaping with food ultimately created more stress. In fact, it added a whole new burden to his plate.

Feeling frustrated and discouraged by his weight gain and routinely getting out of breath trying to keep up with his kids, Tom knew of only one way to manage the aftermath of overeating. Twice a year, Tom would follow a strict detox diet for about a month, typically losing up to twenty pounds by drastically cutting calories and subsisting mainly on protein shakes. This would bring down some of his weight, but it never changed the habit of turning to food to escape the stress of life.

This cycle of overeating and undereating became its own kind of habit. It turned into a system that Tom believed "worked" for him to deal with extra weight, an approach that afforded him the chance to go back to overeating so long as he trusted the weight could eventually be lost again.

Yet entering midlife seemed to make everything harder. The effect of eating too much was no longer just the weight gain, but also chronic heartburn, fatigue, and a loss of confidence. In his earlier years, Tom loved to hike with his buddies, but as overeating became more of a habit, he felt too out of shape to join his friends. He was also embarrassed to go to the community pool with his boys, reluctant to reveal his body in a swimsuit.

When Tom and I first spoke, he told me that he responded well to detox diets and considered this a successful approach. But what followed a "successful" month of detoxing for Tom was always many more months of overeating. Usually, Tom regained even more weight as the cycle progressed. It makes perfect sense, too, given that restricting calories and eliminating foods only works by using willpower. Tom's tactic was to restrict and push through his desire for food. Resisting desire only increases it, so once Tom's willpower waned after a month of dieting, the desire to eat resurfaced even stronger, leading Tom to consume even more of the food he loved.

Tom's approach consistently led to weight gain and reinforced more urges to overeat. Psychologically, it did more harm than good, since the less Tom was able to keep off the weight he lost, the more discouraged he felt. During our consultation together, Tom described feeling exhausted by the perpetual hamster wheel of dieting and overeating.

On the spectrum of the emotional appetite, Tom's tendency was to use food as an escape hatch from life. Overeating took the edge off stress and provided momentary relief. It was a reprieve from the demands of his everyday life and an alternative to prioritizing himself. Turning to food distracted Tom from work and disguised itself as "me time." As an escape from pressure of all kinds, overeating relieved him from the exhausting cycle of using willpower on his annual diets.

Once we identified this pattern and Tom recognized the role food played in his life, we could think of Tom's underlying need for relief. Turning to food not only relieved him from the stress of an overpacked schedule, but it also gave him a reprieve from overly restrictive diets. It was a habit that created the opposite effect of what he most desired.

Core Belief: *I deserve a treat.*

A common thought for Tom—and for people who regularly use food to escape—is *I deserve a treat.* Tom learned from an early age that food can be a reward. Candy was given out as prizes, his family took trips to McDonald's after a sports competition, and sometimes his parents took him to a pizza dinner for a good report card. These experiences reinforced the idea in Tom's brain that he was entitled to a treat when he worked hard at something.

But rewarding himself with food was a lousy prize when it came with the physical discomfort of bloat, indigestion, and guilt around overeating. My question for Tom was: How do you really deserve to feel when you've accomplished something?

I taught Tom that the need to escape with eating and reward himself for all his hard work could be changed by reconnecting to himself and what he needs to feel his best. When Tom was in the regular habit of putting himself last, seeking "me time" with food was an easy outlet. Without the energy or awareness to make an intentional decision, overeating reinforced a cycle of neglecting himself and increasing his desire to eat.

Key Mindset Shift: *I want to make time for myself to decompress without food.*

Tom's emotional appetite to escape with food was directly related to sacrificing his own needs and continually overcommitting himself to other things. Powering through work and family obligations and always putting himself on the back burner was a recipe for the desire to overeat. By simultaneously resisting his emotions and overriding his body's natural language, he exhausted himself and diminished the bandwidth to handle urgency around eating. By the time he came up for air and finally made time for himself, his sense of entitlement for food was strong.

When he noticed this habit in action, he began realizing how he ignored his body, making it hard to stay conscious around food. His body had a genuine desire to be well rested, and when he learned how to honor that, there was less of an impulse to escape. When he balanced time for himself with commitments to other people and things, he stayed connected to his body and naturally felt better without eating more.

Key Emotional Shift: From Overwhelmed to Curious

It's easy and familiar to feel overwhelmed and then numb that feeling with food, which is why the habit becomes so insidious for people who escape by eating. Once you identify the pattern, from a place of curiosity you can think about what you truly need. Escaping through overeating happens as the result of overriding your basic needs. When you acknowledge what those needs are—maybe for you, it's more rest or having more fun—you can think about how to satisfy those needs from a place of compassion with yourself.

It's understandable why you might have frequent urges to eat throughout the day if your life feels unbearable. Even work you enjoy, or responsibilities you gladly accept, can be a source of stress when there is an imbalance of self-care. To understand your language of escape with food, it helps to take a compassionate view of yourself. Of course, many of us shift into judging ourselves instead of being kind and compassionate. Notice the difference between the atmosphere judgment creates versus compassion.

Judgment is harsh, critical, and punitive. It makes us feel worse instead of better. It tears us down instead of building us up. It shuts down understanding or curiosity and divides a situation into the moral value of either right or wrong. Many of us are good at judging, whereas practicing self-compassion takes more intention and practice.

Think of a compassionate parent comforting a child when they are upset. Compassion creates an atmosphere of safety and diffuses tension. It helps restore peace, fosters connection, and makes it easier to accept our humanness. You might be thinking that if you're always compassionate, somehow you'll never learn. But the opposite is true.

Judging yourself works to divide you against yourself. It separates the side that wants an escape from food from the side that wants to change the habit. It takes you out of integrity with the whole you, primitive urges and all. Guess what happens when you are out of integrity or alignment with your full self? There is often more rebellion and less interest in wanting to care for yourself. If you're at odds with yourself, there is less motivation to care and support yourself.

So, how to shift from judgment to compassion? Just like shifting gears on a car, it doesn't work to make a dramatic leap between opposite thoughts. If you try to replace a thought like *You have no self-control* with one like *You are totally confident around food*, but it's not believable, you'll be met with a lot of resistance from your brain. You'll create more mental tension instead of less. An easier place to land, and a more comfortable place to settle in your thinking, is by shifting into neutral to start.

Neutral thoughts and feelings tend to feel easier to accept and are a good way to gradually evolve your beliefs. Before you can get to a compassionate view, a neutral view might look like acknowledging the facts of what you ate. Let's imagine you grazed on cheese, crackers, wine, and chocolate for a few hours. The judgmental view might sound like *You have no self-control*, while the neutral view is more like *You ate cheese, crackers, and chocolate and had some wine*. See how the neutral perspective takes an opinion out of the equation and simply states what is. From this vantage point, it's not a matter of good, bad, right, or wrong but just the facts of what took place.

A neutral response creates a more open space to consider and be curious about yourself. The possibilities of what you can choose to think about a neutral circumstance broaden and are less extreme than either/or beliefs. You get to decide what you want to make overeating mean, and letting go of judgment toward yourself eases negative emotions.

One of best antidotes to escapism with food is bringing yourself back to the power inside right now. Getting lost in the overwhelm of everything on your "to-do" list comes from focusing outside of what you have control over in the present moment. But the overwhelm itself can serve as a kind of tap on the shoulder to bring you back to the here and now.

The Process

1. Identify the pattern of escaping in your everyday life. When does it usually happen and under what circumstances? How are you usually feeling in that situation before you have the urge to eat?

2. Plan for the next time you're in this situation. Write down what food you will eat based on the meals you need to satisfy your hunger and satiety cues. Then also buffer in breaks in your schedule, even if just for five to ten minutes to give yourself a break. It could be sitting back in your chair and closing your eyes while connecting with your breath. Or it might be getting outside for some fresh air. The idea is to carve out space to connect with yourself, recenter how you feel, and calm yourself through your breathing.

3. Recognize the emotion you're experiencing by labeling it without judgment. This simple act is the first step to processing how you feel without eating. By doing this, you acknowledge and make space for that feeling to exist instead of numbing it with food.

4. If you have the urge to eat, breathe into that urgent feeling and remind yourself that it's OK to feel that way. Tell yourself, "There is nothing I need to do right now except breathe and relax into my body."

5. When it's time for your meal, make time and space to eat without distractions so you can be fully present with yourself and feel satisfied by the flavor and nourishment of the food.

For Tom, it took writing down and committing to a food plan to uncover the desire to escape with food. In his first month working with me, following the plan was easy because he was motivated and excited by the prospect of losing weight. Things were under control at work, and Tom was confident about both his staff and the company's trajectory. But midway through his coaching program, Tom had a setback. When a corporate project did not work out according to plan, and Tom felt responsible for picking up the slack, he noticed himself showing up in the kitchen unexpectedly.

At this point in our coaching together, Tom had already lost fifteen pounds and was in the regular habit of writing down his daily food plan. Regularly grazing on food throughout the day was not something he did anymore. So it stood out as something unusual when it happened.

During our call, Tom described feeling under pressure to turn things around with his company and take over projects he would normally delegate to employees. Being an overachiever, he was used to taking on work, often at the detriment of his own well-being. It was easier to say yes to things instead of deliberately allowing for white space in his calendar. There is a sense of accomplishment and validation that people like Tom are used to seeking to measure their own success. But in the absence of any downtime, stress and fatigue accumulate, and eating seems like a natural distraction from both.

"I found myself, in between calls for work, standing with my head in the fridge," Tom told me during one of our sessions. "You don't need anything in here, I told myself."

Because of Tom's intentional work of deciding on his meals ahead of time, he knew something was off when he started rummaging through the fridge outside of mealtimes. Without noticing a thought or feeling driving him to get up from his desk and head to the kitchen, Tom was conscious of the old habit once he realized he was looking around for food and was off his plan. This shows how unconscious our relationship with food can be.

The cycle of believing there is too much to do and not enough time comes from scarcity thinking. This default mode of thoughts around "not enough-ness" is tied to your primitive brain's survival mode. Instead of trusting there is enough (time, food, resources, etc.), your brain will opt to think the opposite just to prepare you for the worst. In fact, your brain's negativity bias—automatically assuming the worst-case scenario in most instances instead of the best—will cause it to focus on your situation being dire instead of all good. This tendency assumes that by thinking there is not enough, you might be alerted to potential danger and do what you can to find more. But scarcity thinking almost always disempowers from you.

When you think there is too much to do and not enough time, you probably feel rushed instead of grounded and focused. It puts you into a state of panic or anxiousness, elevates stress levels, and leads to frantic action instead of methodical productivity. When you feel overcommitted and pressed for time, you feel overwhelmed and lack the ability to manage everything you have to do. Instead of feeling empowered, you feel powerless to stay on top of what you have to do.

A natural extension of this sense of powerlessness is eating in a mindless way. Food becomes something that helps you briefly escape the stress, and it's consumed not with deliberateness but with the same frenetic energy you have toward all things in life. The thoughts creating the desire to eat are usually some flavor of "Food will take the edge off," "Eating will help me get through this," or "This is just for me." From this urgent feeling, eating is usually fast while the mind races through all the other things yet to be done.

For someone who escapes with food, eating doesn't provide much long-term relief. Instead of freeing up time and energy, it depletes them. Instead of regaining a sense of confidence and capability, those things lessen as well. The result of overeating for escape is that it just adds one more thing to the proverbial to-do list. Ultimately, there is no escaping the side effects of too much food because the body needs to be reckoned with.

Chronic stress, weight gain, and indigestion can lead to issues with sleep, cardiovascular health, and overall immunity. Instead of helping to achieve what's important, mindless eating ends up making it much harder.

Somewhere in your own history, dear reader, you may have opted to escape a difficult experience or feeling by eating. When you escape with food enough times, the neural pathway between the thought and feeling is so reinforced that it's firmly planted in the subconscious mind. Maybe every time there is the vibration of anxiousness in your body, your brain identifies that it's an emotion usually numbed with food. You may not even realize what's happening, only that you have a strong craving for some chocolate. Your brain, in its effort to be efficient and expend the least amount of energy possible, stores well-practiced thought patterns in the unconscious. Therefore, you may sometimes notice yourself eating without remembering why you made the choice to put food in your mouth. It wasn't from the realization of hunger in your body, but rather an association that you must eat for relief of some kind.

When you stand from a seated position, you don't notice the thought *It's time to stand up*. But there is a thought process happening, spurring you to take action. With food, your well-practiced eating habits start to seem like a way of life—until you choose to plan intentionally what you will eat and when.

On the surface, planning may seem like a set of rules you have to follow. You might relate it to a diet that feels unnatural and tedious to consistently follow. I argue that in the absence of a plan, you are allowing your primitive reflexes to control you instead of the more evolved, strategic part of your brain. The objective of planning is not to impose rules or create a strict regimen that makes your life more challenging. Instead, it's a way to separate the choices you make from intention, based on what you want long-term, from impulsive ones that are emotional instead of rational in nature.

You are making choices either way.

As I mentioned earlier, sometimes a client will rebel against their own plan, thinking, *I don't want anyone telling me what to do.* The question I ask is always "Who is telling you what to do?"

Remember, when you create a plan ahead of time, it is still *you* making decisions for yourself. When you react to an urge in the moment, it is still *you* making the choice. Your habits around eating, depending on whether they are intentional or mindless, will reveal to you who is running the show. If you feel stuck in a cycle of overeating and powerless to stay in control around food, you've probably surrendered to your primitive brain *telling you what to do*. This part of your thinking can sound like a tyrant, demanding and throwing a fit until it gets its way.

When you come up with a plan for yourself, it should be based on what foods will serve you best (depending on your goals) and what you can really commit to. When you're in integrity with yourself, this looks like considering what you want for pleasure and well-being and on what your future self is likely to benefit from.

This is different from a diet in the sense that weight loss is not the point. Losing pounds can be a likely result of following your plan, but the goal is really to bring consciousness back to your relationship with food. When you plan a piece of chocolate, for instance, instead of eating it spontaneously, the experience is much different. Instead of reacting to the urge for the cake, you will likely eat it from a calmer place. It is much easier to stay in control and eat a moderate amount when you are not eating from a sense of urgency or abundant desire.

Food for Thought

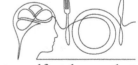

1. Create a personal sanctuary for yourself at home that includes relaxing and revitalizing pleasures. Maybe it's a corner of a room where you have a comfy chair with inspiring reading and a candle nearby. Or it could be an outside area with an inviting view of nature and a wind chime close by.

2. When you might otherwise regularly eat, make it a routine to spend time in that space to practice unwinding without food.

3. The idea is to change the habit of eating to escape and instead proactively relax without food so you can experience the difference of enhanced well-being when you're not overfed.

Chapter 10:

Connection

When Sydney started working with me, she was close to two hundred pounds. She described herself as someone who had always been chubby as a child. When I asked her about the last time she overate, she described a party with friends and a table full of her favorite snacks. There were chips and homemade guacamole, pico de gallo, two different kinds of queso, and a group of graduate students hanging out together on a Saturday afternoon. Appetizers led to an Italian dinner prepared by a private chef and several rounds of drinks.

"I wasn't even hungry by the time dinner rolled around," Sydney admitted as we considered what led her to keep eating. "But everyone was having a good time, and it was all just part of the experience."

Food was the bond Sydney had with her friends. It created a shared experience.

Sydney is not alone in thinking that eating helps her belong and makes it easier to connect to friends and loved ones. Communing over food is a ritual we've all practiced to some degree or another since the beginning of life. It is a way we spend time together and share in the mutual necessity of nourishing our bodies. Connecting over food is not what led Sydney to feel frustrated with her body. It was overeating food, beyond what her body needed at its ideal size, that affected her in an adverse way.

What led Sydney to put another guac-laden chip in her mouth, or say yes to another round of martinis when she already felt comfortably full?

Simple: Everyone else was doing it, and she was part of the collective experience.

It felt awkward for Sydney to stand empty-handed around her friends or turn down a cocktail when everyone else was imbibing. "I didn't want to seem weird," she told me. "It's just what we do together."

Over the course of our coaching sessions, connecting with people in the absence of abundant food and alcohol proved to be the predominant challenge for Sydney. When she was going through the motions of day-to-day work and home life, Sydney easily stuck to her food plan and felt both satisfied and confident. The challenge arose around her social life—meeting up with colleagues for drinks, attending a group dinner, or showing up to a gathering where food and alcohol were abundant. Sydney's main thought in these situations was "I don't want people to think I'm weird."

Connection, and belonging to the group, traces back to our caveman days when survival was more likely if we stayed part of the pack. Separating from the tribe threatened our ability to thrive as people. Our brain has not evolved beyond this need. The primitive brain is still motivated by the need to stay connected.

It's true that not partaking in the collective eating or drinking may cause people to judge you. Feeling disconnected and judged only happens when we a) think it's true and b) decide that it matters. Consider that overeating actually lessens a deep connection between people because it's a distraction from being present and attentive. If you want to test this theory, simply put your fork down during the duration of your next conversation and focus all your attention on listening to the other person.

When you are less focused on food, you may be more connected to yourself and the person you're with. This can make it seem uncomfortable in a different way, separate from being judged or rejected by others. When you are present with yourself and truly in the moment while relating to another person, food no longer disguises the truth. There is a heightened awareness of reality, of who people are and the nature of a situation, unfiltered by the collective haze of overeating and drinking. You may discover that the people you thought were fun and interesting are less appealing when you don't have a taquito in your mouth. Or that an event leaves much to be desired without an open bar to sidle up to.

To Sydney's credit, she tested the experience of maintaining her active social life without always eating and drinking her way through it. Like many people I work with who use food to connect, Sydney was wary of her ability to follow through on an intentional eating and drinking plan.

"People know me as someone who drinks," she told me. "They will wonder why I'm not."

Core Belief: *I might stand out if I don't join in.*

When eating is how you connect with people, it can easily lead to indulging beyond what feels comfortable and satisfying for your body. Eating to be part of the collective experience is a type of FOMO (Fear of Missing Out) characterized by wanting to be part of the group. It shows up especially at cocktail hour, dinner parties, potlucks, buffets, extended afternoon soirees, and any other event that involves socializing with food and beverage in hand.

Sometimes the experience involves a mindset of deliberately overindulging in a mindless way, and if you're not going along with the group vibe, you may be called out. People who relate to this not only feel the need to eat or drink to be accepted, but they often believe they need to adopt the group thinking that goes along with it. Showing restraint while everyone else in attendance is heedlessly consuming makes someone like Sydney feel isolated or set apart. It is not just the eating that matters, but also the attitude of carelessness that helps people trying to connect feel assimilated.

Key Mindset Shift: *I can only control my own happiness.*

To lower your emotional appetite for connection, you need to shift from meeting other people's expectations to serving your own. This will likely feel uncomfortable at first as you wade into the territory of potentially disappointing others. So that you don't disappoint yourself, remember that you can't control how

other people feel through your actions. Other people are responsible for themselves. Ensuring your own happiness requires
committing to a new way of showing up.

When you have a large emotional appetite for connection,
some of your usual thoughts that create desire to eat may include:

- *I don't want to let anyone down.*
- *People will think I'm weird.*
- *I will draw attention to myself.*

Shifting your mindset requires identifying those old beliefs
and observing them if they pop up again. Acknowledge these
thoughts as part of the old habit instead of the truth. You can
ignore those suggestions from your brain just like you would
a broken record playing the background. Instead, connect back
to yourself and notice how your body feels. Remind yourself, *I
can only control my own happiness*, and stay empowered and
connected to your own authority.

Key Emotional Shift: From Obligated to Committed

When you use overeating to connect with people, it's usually
from a feeling of obligation. Perhaps it's an obligation to go with
the flow and blend in so you're not ostracized by the group. You
abandon your body's natural signals telling you it's not hungry
and that you've already had enough, and you dismiss yourself
in the process. Feeling committed to yourself happens when you
remember that only you control your own happiness. You are
always in charge of yourself, and you have the power to make
choices in your best interest.

When you turn to food for a sense of belonging, reconnecting with yourself in the absence of food feels unnatural at first. You need to learn the unfamiliar terrain of your body through its physical and emotional language. Then, over time, it becomes a familiar, safe space. You can relearn how to make connecting to yourself the most natural thing in the world. To be at home with yourself is where a sense of belonging and safety is found, through the door of your feelings that rise when you make room for them.

The Process

1. Decide what kind of experience is important for you to have. Think about what you want to eat and drink by imagining your future self and feeling your best in the moment.

2. Write down a plan of what you will eat and drink, considering any obstacles that might arise and visualizing yourself handling the urge to go off plan.

3. Think about what you will say if you need to turn down extra food or alcohol and rehearse it in advance. Keep it short and simple. Write it down somewhere where you can refer to it later, and also jot down what thoughts will inspire you to stay committed to yourself.

4. Consider how you want to feel at the end of the day, and the comfort you will have in your body and mind. Imagine that in advance.

5. If you eat and drink off plan, be sure to reflect on what happened before you go to sleep that evening. Bring awareness to the thinking that led you to abandon your

plan so you can identify underlying patterns in your thoughts and actions and then learn from the experience.

Sydney scheduled an outing to a winery with friends, and a week before the date the two of us hashed out a plan. We considered whether Sydney wanted to eat or drink, how much, and any obstacles that might hinder her ability to follow her plan. She was apprehensive that she could stick to her goal, even though it's what she wanted.

This didn't surprise me. Sydney, like many people who are used to connecting over food, based her identity on past experiences with friends and the image of herself always drinking and going with the flow of the collective experience. When Sydney thought about going to the winery, she felt anxious despite having a plan laid out for what she wanted to eat and drink. During our coaching session, Sydney was clear that she wanted to pass on drinking wine and opt for coffee instead. She perused the food menu in advance and decided on a mixed greens salad with blue cheese, walnuts, and dried figs.

Sydney felt some apprehension about committing to her plan. She didn't yet see herself as someone who doesn't drink wine at wineries, and she wasn't sure she could do it. This is normal since the brain refers to past experience as evidence of what is possible. Sydney did not yet have evidence that she could successfully eat and drink less when out with friends. So, she used her plan and leaned into the possibility that it was possible for her to do it. She even visualized herself ahead of time being around her friends and staying committed to her plan. All this helped strengthen Sydney's commitment to follow through.

When I touched base with Sydney on our next call, I learned that she successfully stuck to the plan—and it was easier than she anticipated. Despite the warning from her brain, Sydney was relieved to find that her friends cared less than she thought about what Sydney chose to eat and drink. In fact, one friend was inspired by Sydney's decision to pass on alcohol.

Many of my clients, after seeing what life is like with less alcohol, decide they don't miss it as much as they expected. Once a new routine is established and they feel the benefits of fewer cravings, better sleep, more energy, and clearer focus, the advantages to unwinding with a cocktail or glass of wine diminish. There is less desire for a drink when the desire to feel good outweighs it. Desire is repurposed to experiencing the natural pleasure that comes with well-being.

For another portion of my clients, having alcohol in their life is still important. Together, we develop an intentional plan for how the pleasure of a drink can be enjoyed mindfully. Feeling empowered to drink in moderation is a skill we can teach ourselves once we understand how to handle urges more effectively. Sydney is an example of a client who appreciated not drinking most of the week but also savored opportunities when she could deliberately imbibe with friends.

Sydney preferred to pass on drinking during her day-to-day routine as a graduate student, but once a month or so, she chose to engage in the collective experience of several rounds of drinks with friends. She explained to me that relating to her friends during an extended afternoon of watching football or hanging out on the lawn at the school campus meant being in the same frame of mind. Planning several drinks for Sydney was as much about being part of the collective mindset of her friends as it was about enjoying the taste of alcohol.

"It's a different experience when you're the only sober one," Sydney explained to me on one of our calls.

Occasionally being part of the collective drinking experience was valuable to Sydney. Participating in several rounds of cocktails and interacting with her friends in that same mindset was a type of fun she desired, at least during this season of her life. To stay in the habit of making thoughtful choices, based on what she really wanted (instead of what other people or society wanted for her), Sydney evaluated what made those types of experiences pleasurable. She considered how she could maximize the overall fun, both in the moment and afterward.

What worked was deciding ahead of time on what she would drink and how much. She also planned what she would eat, knowing it can be easy to over-snack when she's less inhibited. This is how Sydney stayed in control of her eating and drinking without giving up the desire to be part of the collective experience.

The process of unraveling the habit of connecting with food requires learning how to reconnect with yourself. Being willing to explore the uncharted territory of your inner desire and respond more to your body than to other people is a process that takes time and practice. Every opportunity of advocating for yourself instead of following the group is a chance to build confidence in your ability to connect and take care of yourself.

When you don't follow your plan perfectly, you have a chance to better understand the thought and habit driving your desire to eat. If you're able to set aside frustration or disappointment with yourself, you're more able to accept and understand yourself at a deeper level. Nothing has gone wrong when the old habit of choosing others over yourself pops back up again. Your past self has spent many years believing you need to eat more to belong. It will take some time to solidify your new identity as someone who prioritizes himself or herself first and pays close attention to the inner language of the body instead of the suggestions of other people.

Food for Thought

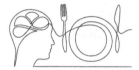

1. Before a special event when you might be tempted to overeat, spend time imagining yourself at the event in a way that you successfully navigate all the obstacles and follow your ideal plan. The power of visualization doesn't need to be reserved only for Olympic athletes. By picturing your future self showing up with confidence and authority around food, you can create a mental imprint or muscle memory of taking that same action.

2. Come up in advance with the steps you will take in this challenging situation so you are more prepared.

3. Map out a mental plan of the ways to pivot and adapt should obstacles pop up along the way. Visualization will help you anticipate problems ahead of time and strategize so you're set up for success.

4. Take note of what happened at the actual event. What was the result of the visualizing and preparing you did?

Chapter 11:

Pleasure

When I worked as a sous chef at a high-end resort, I thought I'd reached the pinnacle of success. My first stint in fine dining involved spending hours peeling the delicate skin off yellow tomatoes to turn into a golden sorbet. Then I mastered the art of dicing piles of red onions into purple cubed *brunoise* that fit perfectly on a demitasse spoon. At another restaurant I was taught that fingerling potato puree is not velvety until each tiny tuber is methodically peeled, boiled, and passed through a ricer to remove any hidden lumps. And most memorably, I learned how to sculpt cases of tough, fibrous artichokes into smoothly carved hearts that could be folded into risotto.

This painstaking work took extra time—hours not always allocated under a tightly controlled payroll. This meant that sometimes I worked for free. I often skipped breaks and grabbed spoonfuls or pieces of food to cobble together sustenance as

I worked. It demanded a physical intensity that sent spasms through my back and caused my hands to clench into tight fists as I slept. Each morning, I woke up to the painful job of gently uncurling my fingers from bound-up tendons inflamed from repetitive motion.

I willingly did this year after year because I had an insatiable passion for food. My appetite for success in the professional kitchen was driven by an obsession to elevate everyday ingredients into full-blown rapture. And while the work involved the service, feeding, and care of outside diners, my drive was entirely self-serving. I wanted to satisfy my own voracious hunger.

It was selfish. It was indulgent. It made complete sense to me.

Balancing Pleasure: More Is Not Always Better

Humans are wired to seek pleasure. The reward center of our brains recognizes pleasure from food, and the dopamine released motivates us to eat again. This is part of our primal instinct to survive, because without the motivation to eat, we would starve. Before man manipulated food into processed ingredients, humans ate natural, whole foods: protein and dairy from animals and plants, vegetables from the earth, and natural sugars from fruits and honey. These whole foods, full of fiber, digest more slowly in the body and release a small hit of dopamine from the pleasure center of the brain.

Processing natural ingredients such as sugarcane and wheat into refined substances both expedites their absorption into the body and concentrates the reward we experience in the brain. Instead of a moderate amount of dopamine, when we eat something with granulated sugar, we experience an intense surge of the feel-good chemicals. Our brains mistakenly assume that sugar must be good for our survival since it creates so much dopamine. Through thoughts created in our brain, we believe we need even more sugar, even though more sugar does not equate with better chances of survival. That primal part of the brain was not designed to handle the effect of man-made food or concentrated ingredients produced from natural foods.

Like drugs that create a temporary high, certain foods produce pleasure by triggering the reward center of the brain. As with drugs, the brain does not differentiate this intense pleasure from what helps us thrive as humans and what does not. In response to the dopamine surge we get from eating food, our brain encourages us to have more. That's why it can feel hard to stop after one bite of cake or a few sips of wine. It's not because you lack willpower or self-control; it's because your brain is responding to its well-designed reward center.

The goal is not to eliminate pleasure or make food boring, but rather to enhance the overall pleasure you experience in life. If you're someone who uses food as your primary source of pleasure, notice how the pleasure diminishes with every additional bite. When your emotional appetite drives you to seek more food, it limits the pleasure felt in your body, the pleasure of your emotional health, the pleasure of utilizing your mind, and the pleasure from engaging deeply with others.

Where is pleasure felt? Our five senses are receptors, and when we eat, we engage all of them when we are fully conscious. Yet mindless eating, done in response to a primitive impulse, is the opposite of conscious eating. It's reacting to a feeling, whether desire or disappointment, that leads us to eat to feel better. Reactive eating, instead of intentional eating, robs us of all the pleasure to be had from food.

Your brain wants to capitalize on pleasure. It mistakenly thinks more must be better. Therefore, the idea of having a glass of wine and some chips *while* watching a movie on Netflix and lying in a comfy bed seems like such a good idea. People with an emotional appetite for pleasure often add eating and drinking to other experiences to make the experience even more amazing— as if layering on dopamine from multiple sources will heighten the enjoyment and maximize the pleasure. You can't have too much of a good thing, right?

Usually there is momentary pleasure from eating something delicious. There's no denying that. But when you consider the longer view—not necessarily the long-term view but the view a couple of hours after overeating for pleasure—the effect is much different. When you obey repeated urges for food and mindlessly eat beyond what your body comfortably needs, it creates diminished pleasure on the other side of momentary pleasure. For some people, it's feeling an even stronger desire to go back for second helpings and less empowerment to stop eating. There is a hangover effect of guilt, indigestion, and an inability to enjoy other natural pleasures without food and alcohol coming to the party. There can be a reckoning first thing the next morning, a type of awareness that this doesn't sit well with you physically and psychologically. It's the opposite of well-being or continued pleasure.

What I've discovered through my own journey and helping clients with this work is that there is a tipping point with pleasure. Once you know this, you can find your personal sweet spot where you maximize the pleasure found in food while optimizing feeling the best you can in your body.

We all desire different kinds of pleasure; the trick is to balance and prioritize them in a way that creates long-term well-being and satisfaction. For my clients, the pleasures they want are usually enjoyment of food, feeling comfortable in their own skin, the ease of dressing and wearing clothes they love, confidence and authority over their choices, pride in their appearance, agility and strength in their body, having fun, feeling relaxed, physical comfort, and trusting themselves. These things are not incompatible—meaning you don't need to give up one to have another. But it does require some understanding of your brain and how to stay alert to its sneaky suggestions.

The first point of awareness is often once you realize that too much of a good thing is causing consequences that limit your pleasure and enjoyment. When you continue to eat past physical satisfaction, it's usually for emotional reasons. The reason may be as straightforward as just wanting to experience the taste and mouthfeel of something delicious. This is desiring pleasure for pleasure's sake—except that pleasure from food doesn't continue to grow the more you consume.

It's the first bite or sip of something that reveals its full flavor. Taste buds are most sensitive to the nuances in taste when they aren't dulled by other ingredients we've eaten. It's also true that when you're responding to a strong feeling of desire or the strong urge to eat, you're likely to consume your food faster. The faster you eat, the less likely you are to savor and relish the full experience of a meal.

The full experience is more than just tasting, chewing, and swallowing, which is what it can seem like when you're inhaling food instead of being mindful of each bite. But each bite can potentially satisfy more than just the sense of taste. When you take time to appreciate the aesthetic of your food, either through the colors and shapes on the plate, or even the beauty of the serving dish itself, it delights your sense of sight. This pleasure in enjoying food by how it looks can be satisfying when you pay attention to it. Pausing to notice the visual appeal of your meal also initiates a mindful approach to your eating. From there, you are more likely to consider the first bite with intention and thoughtfulness.

With the first bite, there are more senses to notice and contemplate. Perhaps the initial sensation is the feel of food on your lips and tongue. Is it cold, hot, or lukewarm? Maybe it has the contrast of different temperatures if you're eating a slice of warm apple pie with cold vanilla ice cream on top. There might be layers of texture, too. Smooth and creamy along with chewy and crisp may be sensed if you're slowing down and considering the way food feels in your mouth. This type of focused perception is what many of us override when we're driven by the urge to eat and do it quickly. We respond impulsively and with the fast energy that comes from thinking, *I just want it*.

The key to stopping is knowing how to stay connected to your body while eating. When you're practiced at listening to your inner language with its cues of hunger and fullness, you'll discover when your body responds with "enough" in its own way. Maybe it's sensed by a pause between bites and pushing your chair away from the table. Perhaps it's a shift in your stomach when the sensation of hunger disappears. Or you may clearly hear a thought in your mind telling you, "We're good." The more you listen, recognize, and honor those cues, the more aware you will be. It will feel comfortable, more habitual, to stop at that sweet spot.

But how do you determine where that sweet spot is when you're just a beginner?

What most of us are familiar with is using portion size as a measure of how much we need to eat. This visual cue takes the focus off your body's internal cue, but it's a fine starting point when you're beginning to discover your sweet spot.

Core Belief: *More is better.*

When you are more focused on the pleasure of food than the wellness of your body there is a mistaken assumption that more food equates to higher satisfaction. Since you are paying more attention to the food in front of you it's easy to miss the subtle cues from your body telling you it has had enough. Believing more food leads to more pleasure drives you to eat beyond what is truly satisfying to your food and perpetuates the habit of stopping at fullness instead of at a point of "just enough." The awareness kicks in once you notice the discomfort settle in from overeating. At that point you can intellectually connect the dots that more food is ultimately less pleasurable when you consume it with disregard for your body.

Key Mindset Shift: *This is more than enough to be fully satisfied.*

When your emotional appetite is for pleasure, and more of it, you need to train your brain that more is not better. You can anticipate that if you're around your favorite food or something delicious, you might notice either the suggestion to keep eating or the feeling or urgency to put more into your mouth. The mindset shift is reminding yourself that the portion you decided on is more than enough and be willing to notice the suggestion for more without acting on it.

Key Emotional Shift: From Dismissive to Satisfied

If you abandon your food plan once you're physically satisfied and keep eating from the urge for more, you're dismissing the cue of satiety coming from your body. You might notice that the hunger is gone and your body is subtly saying, "That's enough," but you dismiss these signs because you think more is better. To change this habit and teach yourself that following your plan is better (because you honor your body and eat the appropriate food for satiety), you need to recognize the feeling of being dismissive or the urgency for more and be curious about it instead of mindlessly reacting to it. Going from dismissive to curious requires noticing either the suggestion or feeling motivating you to want more and observing that experience as it happens. It helps to expect the feeling to occur in your body and anticipate it happening so you can be vigilant while eating.

The Process

1. Make a plan to eat when you're hungry and include foods that nourish and satisfy you.

2. As part of this plan, be specific that you will eat two spoonfuls less at each meal.

3. If your brain suggests, "That's not enough," remind yourself that it's "plenty."

4. Eat slowly, paying attention to the sensory experience of each bite, and notice what happens to the hunger in your body.

5. Stop when you've finished your portion—or before if you notice any of the signs that hunger is gone and you've reached satiety.

6. Be curious about how your body feels right then, an hour later, and after four hours. Consider what's different in the way your body feels when it's lighter. If hunger returns after an hour, eat just enough to take the edge off that hunger.

7. If it's your last meal of the day, also pay attention to how your body feels first thing the next morning.

When you're discovering your personal sweet spot, you want to notice when the amount of eating and drinking starts to have an adverse reaction on how well you feel in your body and mind. For instance, maybe having two cookies allows you to experience enough pleasure without the discomfort of indigestion, fatigue, or any other unpleasant side effect. But when you have more, you notice the aftermath offsets the pleasure of eating.

Especially with processed foods (mainly manufactured snacks or anything with flour, sugar, or alcohol), you will notice an increase in cravings for these foods the more you eat or drink.

The sweet spot lies in your ability to eat an ideal amount of these foods so the desire to eat more is minimized. Cravings and the mental chatter of wanting more of those foods disrupt the please and ease of losing weight and maintaining your ideal body.

For me, having some chocolate a few times a week is satisfying and pleasurable because I've determined the sweet spot of including it in my regular way of eating. But I don't have it every day because I know it might increase my desire and the habitual need to have it, which is unpleasant.

When it comes to wine, I've mastered having two glasses along with a single portion of dessert once a week. The negative impact on these choices is minimal, and I can easily forego alcohol and desserts the rest of the week. But when I indulge in drinking multiple nights of the week, the pull for more is stronger.

That doesn't mean you can't plan for more indulgences. There are times over the holidays or when I'm traveling when I decide to drink or eat more. But my well-thought-out plan anticipates that when I resume my usual way of eating, there will likely be a temporary period of more cravings. There will be an adjustment phase of eating and drinking less of the processed foods, and I don't make that discomfort either a problem or a reason to eat more.

To get back to the sweet spot of less hunger and cravings for extra food, you need to go through a short period of allowing the discomfort of more urges until your body and brain adjusts.

A Note on Drinking and Pleasure

Imagine a series of dots being connected in your brain. That's what it's like for those neural pathways. Like water flowing along a riverbed, the chain reaction of your thoughts and feelings follows the well-worn grooves of the habits you've practiced. After you've consented to buying your favorite wine, the act of drinking it starts to manifest. Maybe all that remains is the right set of circumstances, thoughts, and feelings, and you find yourself cracking open the bottle one Friday evening. It could be after a particularly hard day at work, or because you had a difficult conversation with a friend. If you're someone who typically pours a drink when you feel anxious, your brain may just wait for that familiar emotion to vibrate in your body before quickly reminding you about the wine in the house.

It's an efficient way for your brain to return to the dopamine reward it desires. Once you take the time to disconnect each dot in the habit and recognize what's at the heart of your desire, the pattern can be changed. To use the example of feeling anxious, having a drink can dull the vibration of that emotion in your body. It numbs the sensation created in your nervous system and is like a pleasurable dulling of the tension anxiousness creates. You might believe having a drink relaxes you or takes the edge off. The more you continue using alcohol—or food for that matter—to feel better when you're anxious, the more often that urge will appear when you're anxious. It's not that pouring yourself a drink to relax is a problem; it's just a question of whether you always want to use alcohol as a way to get some relief.

How well does drinking solve anxiousness?

If for you, it's consuming some chips or a bowl of ice cream, swap that for the alcohol in this example. How well does the food or alcohol truly help you relax and feel better?

My personal journey of drinking less wine evolved over time. When I worked professionally as a chef, drinking a couple glasses of wine in the evening seemed like par for the course. The study of wine is considered by many culinary professionals to be an art in and of itself and a worthy pursuit of one's time. It is widely believed that wine enhances the flavor of food, and as you can tell by this point, I am all about increasing the pleasure of food. In my twenties and thirties, there were plenty of reasons why I didn't question drinking wine every evening.

You already know how things changed when I turned forty. Food and alcohol started affecting me in different ways. While wine relaxed me momentarily, I started to notice the ways it also made my life harder. When I started to think intentionally about food, it made sense to also consider my choices around drinking wine. I'm using the example of wine here because it was the drink I desired most on a regular basis.

In those early days of rethinking my habits with drinking, I began by making choices ahead of time regarding how much to drink. I practiced giving myself days without drinking to notice what life was like without it. I approached my planning with food and wine like a scientist conducting research, or a chef experimenting with a new recipe. I was curious to see how I felt when food and wine were no longer helping me relax. I didn't have any intention of giving up wine, as I still held tightly to my enjoyment of it, but I also wanted to see whether limiting it would alleviate the negative effects I often experienced afterward.

This process really helped to show me the difference between my experience after a couple glasses of wine and my experience without it. In that space of being curious about how life was different with and without wine, I could evaluate the advantages and disadvantages of including it in my life. One thing I noticed on the days I drank was that I felt tired within an hour of finishing a glass of wine. My energy was zapped, it was difficult to focus or engage in things I liked to do in the evening, and I just wanted to crawl into bed. Sleep came quickly but didn't last long. Usually about three hours into my slumber, the downside of drinking set in, and anxious thoughts streamed through my mind more often than not.

Sleep eluded me on nights after two glasses of wine. When I finally settled back into sleep after lying awake for hours, there wasn't enough time to rest before waking. Days after drinking were noticeably foggier, too. It seemed to take twice as much coffee before I felt alert, and even then, I noticed dulled thinking and drudgery around completing daily tasks. Urges for food increased on these days, too. Then the desire to take the edge off with another glass of wine felt even stronger.

Still, my reasons to keep drinking were strong. While I was ready to pay attention to the experience of having wine in a new way, I was not ready to give it up completely.

It really helped me to use this approach to changing the habit.

Instead of going all in on regular drinking with thoughts like *It doesn't matter, Everybody does it, This is normal, Wine is healthy,* or *Wine makes everything better,* I gave myself a pause in the habit to consider life on the other side. I was curious without swearing it off all together.

It's tempting to buy into the brain's extremist tendency and go all or nothing with alcohol. You may decide it's necessary to banish drinking completely from your life. As with certain kinds of food, maybe you learned that alcohol is "bad" or a poison that you really shouldn't include in your life. But equally as challenging to negotiate is the social and cultural pressure we are fed daily that drinking is normal, fun, sophisticated, and even healthy. Both sides of the equation can seem true at times, and instead of deciding based on what other people believe is right, your relationship with alcohol is your own to navigate.

A problem for some people who swear off drinking completely is that alcohol becomes a forbidden fruit. Making it off limits can increase your desire for it. This is problematic not just because it can set you up to want it more. When you think you shouldn't drink and believe it's wrong to occasionally partake, it creates a heavy burden if one day you go against yourself and indulge. Then, as someone who imbibed in a "bad" substance, you might judge yourself as bad or wrong and spiral into a place of shame.

But like food, alcohol doesn't have any moral value. It's one of many beverage options that just sits there. It's your thoughts about it that determine the experience you have with it.

For me, thinking *You will never have that again* brought up feelings of deprivation and resentment. It felt like something was being taken away from me, and it only made me want it more. It wasn't a useful thought if my goal was to want wine less instead of more.

The trajectory of my relationship with wine looks like a downward sloping line. It started out consistently high, with me drinking a couple glasses of wine every night. Then, after experimenting with drinking 50 percent less, I chose to take a break from drinking completely for about six months. That six-month hiatus taught me a lot that served me in my eventual relationship with alcohol and in my approach to food. When wine wasn't part of my weekly plan, or a weekend add-on, I stopped caring about it as much. My routine changed, and I stopped anticipating it. I no longer felt like every Friday afternoon was a countdown to five o'clock when I could finally cork open a new bottle of wine.

That was a huge benefit of staying sober for a longer stretch. Anyone who regularly drinks understands the pull alcohol can have and the antsy feelings of needing it to take the edge off at the end of the day. When that edge disappeared, I felt a lovely sense of freedom. Sleep became more regular, my moods stabilized, a glow fell over my complexion, and general aches and pains diminished.

It was hard to argue against these improvements in favor of the chance to restart wine time. But it turns out that the dopamine flood from alcohol is not easily forgotten by the brain. While my need to drink almost completely went away, the flame of desire did not extinguish.

Holidays and dinners out were particularly challenging. "Maybe it would be OK to have a drink this time," my brain whispered occasionally. "It's not a problem to have a drink or two on the weekend."

Somewhere between realizing the negative effects of drinking and taking for granted how well I felt without it, I began entertaining the suggestion from my brain that it wouldn't be a big deal to have a drink from time to time. This wasn't a stretch to agree with because I never totally swore off drinking in the first place.

Reintroducing alcohol began with having a glass of wine here and there with dinner on Saturday or Sunday night. Soon the anticipation resurfaced. Dinners no longer felt satisfying without wine. I grew antsy around 4:00 p.m. when the lull before dinner stretched on. Back were the middle-of-the-night wake-up calls and the groggy Sunday mornings nursing a pot of coffee. The new norm was a drink-free workweek, rewarded with wine on the weekend. The habit was easily ingrained.

The old aftermath of drinking was easily spotted, too. Work felt harder, as even two glasses of wine would lessen my focus. It's understandable that when alcohol affects sleep and disrupted sleep contributes to hormonal imbalance and stress, there is a ripple effect on many areas of life. When more effort goes into maintaining the same routine and stress is elevated, having a drink also seems like an easy solution and the way to smooth out the day. You can see, if you're not already familiar with it yourself, how insidious the cycle is.

When I felt embedded in this habit of drinking every weekend, I didn't like the regret I felt after an evening of having wine with dinner. Not getting a restful night's sleep and ending the weekends exhausted instead of refreshed set me up for harder workweeks. Because of my training and the ongoing work I do with my own coach, I knew the solution lay in better understanding my thinking. I needed to find the thought error motivating me to pour some wine.

The two beliefs I discovered behind the decision to regularly drink on the weekend were:

1. "Wine makes the weekends more enjoyable."
2. "It's not a problem to have a few drinks every now and then."

The way to dismantle these beliefs began with a question I often ask my own brain: "How do you know that's true?"

Wine makes the weekends more enjoyable. There are aspects of this belief that are true. What feels pleasurable about having a glass of wine on a Saturday night include the actual anticipation of it, the taste of the wine, the flavor of wine and food paired together, the initial feel-good euphoria of dopamine, and the subdued sensation of being relaxed. That bucket of pleasure might last for up to three hours.

But I also found evidence that this thought is not true. After two glasses of wine, my energy felt zapped. During our usual Saturday evening movie time as a family, you'd find me dozing on the couch ten minutes into the show. I also noticed an uptick in urges to eat, and after drinking, I might negotiate a bowl of ice cream for myself from a less intentional place of reasoning. With a belly full of dessert and wine, it was hard to enjoy the pleasure of reading before bed, since all I felt like doing was crawling under the sheets until morning. Yet my ability to sleep deeply always felt stifled by alcohol. I might easily drift off for the first few hours, but I always awakened to a restless feeling of anxiousness and indigestion.

Lying awake in the middle of night jolted my awareness. There is nothing like a 2:00 a.m. wake-up call to give you a perspective on life, and wine-drinking evenings almost offered the same message: *This doesn't feel good.*

My intuitive sense liked to surface in that quiet space of darkness when none of the usual distractions of work or family could compete with it. It spoke softly but firmly and advocated for the truth to be heard. Unlike the primitive part of my brain, my intuition never demanded anything from me. It served as a compass, always guiding me back to what felt authentic and true for my best self. When I regularly drank, my voice of intuition was by my side in those midnight hours, often reminding me in a gentle way, *This isn't working for us.*

Maybe this has happened to you, too. Our inner truth is not always easy to act on or accept. While I didn't deny my intuition its say, I often felt like it was too hard to act on its suggestion. The pull toward drinking was strong, and it also felt entangled in my identity. I was raised in a family where evening wine time was a celebrated ritual. My Italian ancestors made wine in their basement. As a chef, I was taught to value drinking to enhance the flavor of food and elevate the dining experience. Dismantling wine from my identity seemed complicated and hard. Pouring a glass of wine every weekend usually felt like the easier option.

This brings us back to the tipping point of pleasure.

Many people who come to me for help reach a place where they can no longer ignore their intuition or the glaring sense that something is not right. And that led me to question the second belief: *It's not a problem to have a few drinks every now and then.* For me, it was the anxiety-fueled nights, irritability with my family, and the sinking realization that my children were being influenced by my regular habit of drinking. It wasn't worth it anymore.

Food for Thought

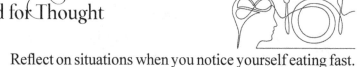

1. Reflect on situations when you notice yourself eating fast. Pay attention to when you begin to feel that quickening pace in your body, which is a sign that you're experi-

encing a desire for more. Sometimes it begins when you visually see food or begin preparing a meal. Your brain senses that food is around, and there are things you enjoy eating, so naturally this creates the desire to eat.

2. Practice connecting to your body and slowing down that urgency by taking a deep breath in and dropping into where you feel the urge. Exhale slowly to calm your nervous system. Deliberately tell yourself, "This is more than enough," to slow down your urgency to eat quickly.

3. When you sit down to eat, practice reconnecting with your body and setting your intention to eat in a slow way. Remind yourself that the portion in front of you is plenty, and the best way to fully enjoy it is by eating slowly and attentively. Allow this to be a slow, tedious process until you get used to eating at a slower pace.

4. If drinking less is your goal, decide exactly how much you want to drink ahead of time, if at all.

5. On your plan, anticipate when you will likely want to drink and how your brain might suggest it to you. Then, when the urge happens, either as a suggestion or a restless feeling, you won't be surprised by it and can just acknowledge, "Oh, this is just an urge, and I can practice sitting in this momentary discomfort until it passes." Remind yourself that you can dismiss the suggestion of a drink and that the experience of sitting in a few minutes of restless energy is not as hard as you think.

Chapter 12:

Learning Your Body's Emotional Language

In chapter 7, I shared Karen's story of unlearning the love language of food. But her journey didn't end with losing weight. Developing a new relationship with both food and herself felt awkward, and in the beginning Karen struggled with believing in her success. It felt strange to see her body quickly transform into a thinner frame while her brain was still associating with her past self. It makes sense, considering she spent most of her life identifying as the "big" one in her family. She spent years and years in a love language with food and letting go of that relationship felt like a loss at first.

During this phase of transition and learning the language of her body, Karen also mourned the loss of food. One of her old go-to ways to connect with her family was in front of the TV, munching on chocolate-covered pretzels. When she began honoring her physical hunger and didn't need the pretzels, it was an opportunity to pay attention to what her body was telling her.

"I feel kind of sad," she told me on one of our calls, "that I'm not eating the pretzels." Karen thought it seemed silly that she would feel this way about snacks, but to me it made perfect sense. She was going through a common phase many of my clients experience: mourning the loss of food. Part of Karen's brain still believed that the pretzels were what created a sense of connection and comfort, and without them, sadness rose to the surface of her body.

Listening to this sadness was part of Karen's process of learning a new language. When food is no longer your love language, you can begin a new dialogue with your body—a dialogue in response to your body's natural language of physical sensations and emotional vibrations. The sensation of hunger, satiety, fatigue, and illness and the vibration of emotions such as sadness, anxiousness, frustration, excitement, and confidence are your body's way of communicating to you information about your life experience. By attentively listening to your body and responding with compassion, you create a new dialogue and language. You begin to love and care for yourself in a more deeply satisfying way.

Sadness didn't feel comfortable to Karen at first. Like many of us who are not used to spending time with emotions, it can seem like a problem that sadness is hanging around. At first, Karen thought there was something wrong with her that she would experience sadness every few days. She asked me how she could get rid of it. She wanted to avoid and resist the sadness, as if it wasn't meant to be there.

But all emotions are valid and worth accepting. They can help you understand yourself and what you're currently thinking about your everyday life. When you resist your emotions, it creates an even more uncomfortable experience. On top of the simple vibration of sadness, you're now dealing with the tension of resistance in trying to keep the sadness at bay.

As Karen learned this new language of her body, she started by identifying what she felt. This is an important first step to validating what your body is communicating to you. She became familiar with the vibration of sadness in her body, which for her felt like a heavy weight at the bottom of her stomach. She also noticed pressure in her throat that radiated out through her chest. The more Karen became familiar with sadness and how it was a natural part of changing her relationship with food, the more easily she could shed the resistance to it.

That tension of resistance, on top of sadness, is like an emotional shield we carry as a way to avoid the discomfort of emotions we're not used to experiencing. The brain interprets emotions like sadness as scary and uncomfortable, and therefore something to be avoided. Some of this is due to the primal brain's natural inclination toward keeping things easy and comfortable and avoiding pain at all costs. But it's also in large part the way many of us were raised: to believe that we shouldn't feel sad or express our emotions. It's common, when we see someone emotionally upset, to immediately respond with "It's OK, calm down" or "Everything's fine; don't worry about it." We unknowingly dismiss others' emotional experiences, reinforcing the belief that we shouldn't feel upset.

This conditioned approach to feelings does nothing to help us work through our emotions and support our bodies. It doesn't help us learn to accept what we're feeling so we can better understand ourselves and know what we deeply value. It makes it easy to lose ourselves and feel disconnected in our relationships with others. When you've lost the sense of your own feelings and what matters to you, it's difficult to be your true self. When you've lost touch with your true self, how can you show up authentically in a relationship with someone else?

When you learn the language of your emotions, however, you create a sense of safety within yourself. You depend less on other people to validate or approve of you, because you're doing it for yourself. Softening the resistance, your body's natural suit of armor, is one of the first steps. I find it helpful to just acknowledge that the resistance is my body's way of trying to protect me from something it perceives as "unsafe." When I recognize that and feel the tightness of resistance around my body, I also start to get curious. I wonder, *What is it that doesn't seem safe for me to feel right now*?

It's OK if you're not sure initially what the deeper emotion is that resistance is trying to block you from experiencing. You can begin by just noticing the resistance itself and teaching yourself how to relax into it. One way to do this is by connecting to your breath, deeply inhaling and exhaling while you release tension. Physically entering in through breath, instead of trying to rationalize how you feel, can be an easier and more immediate way of connecting to your body. Breathing is such a simple and powerful way to calm your nervous system, and the more you practice it, the more you become a master at self-soothing.

Interpreting this new language of your body feels foreign for most food lovers at first. Be willing to practice, without the expectation of trying to solve or get rid of the feeling that's happening in your body. First being aware of the sensation in your body, either from a physical cue or an emotional one, is a powerful first step. This is how you get acquainted with the tapestry of emotions that make up your life. Maybe at first you notice, like I did, that you feel resistance pretty often. This can be a clue that there are other feelings wanting to be heard—feelings that in the past you've always met with resistance.

When I began this work of uncovering the emotional language of my body, I really only identified a handful of feelings I experienced on a weekly basis. Resistance was actually at the top of the list of most frequently felt emotions. Occasionally a feeling like sadness might bubble up, and tears might even come to my eyes out of nowhere, but resistance would quickly descend upon it and shut down the tears.

I was fascinated by this because I had never noticed the habits of my emotions. Until I started paying attention to them, I didn't realize that I usually told myself, "You don't have time for this," whenever sadness spoke up. Unknowingly, I taught myself to be resistant to it. I didn't make the connection to my childhood, when I was told I was "too sensitive," or how I decided back then that it was unacceptable to express how I felt. As children, we don't have the maturity or awareness to understand the validity of our feelings, and we certainly don't have the language to voice what we're going through.

When the belief that feelings are a problem is learned as children and then continued as we age, no wonder many of us food lovers look to escape with eating at any whisper of emotional discomfort.

Many of us reach a point in adulthood when we can no longer deny the language of our body. Your brain may not always be telling the truth when it promises that "food will make you feel better," but your body never lies. The signs of your body's discomfort may be subtle at first, and when you continually pursue a love language with food, you can easily override those signs.

Until you reach the threshold, and you can't.

That's the place many of my clients arrive at when they first reach out to me for help. The tipping point of pain and discomfort in their body surpasses the instant gratification of food. In that moment, when your body says *enough is enough* and you're willing to listen, is often a turning point in your relationship with food. When you're willing to respond to that communication from your body (maybe it's reflux, immobility, pain, or a health crisis) without eating more, it's an opportunity to nurture yourself in a new way.

Paying attention to your body with curiosity and compassion is one way you restore trust with yourself. When you visit your emotions as they appear, it's a chance to establish a sense of safety and security in your body.

As I explored the handful of emotions I noticed at first, I practiced creating a sense of trust by being curious about them instead of judgmental. Many of us have the tendency to think that either we shouldn't be feeling the way we do, or that we should be happier than we are. Both assumptions are a form of rejecting ourselves as well as the truth of what we're experiencing. Instead of accepting ourselves, and the spectrum of natural human emotions that create a rich life experience, we're essentially telling ourselves that it's wrong to feel what we feel. By believing something has gone wrong if we're sad instead of happy, we add emotions like shame, guilt, and resistance on top of the language of sadness. We then make it a harder experience to explore and understand our emotional well-being.

Resistance is sometimes the entry point for many of us to begin letting our guard down with feelings. When I began noticing resistance, it was easy to recognize. It felt tense and constricting, like my muscles were clenching to brace for painful impact. My breathing was often tight and fast, or sometimes I even momentarily held my breath without realizing it—as if I was anticipating something terrible about to happen.

I taught myself how to feel safer exploring the emotions underneath resistance by physically relaxing myself through my breathing. Your breath is a natural entry point into your body and an easy way to access feelings. Remember, feelings are sensations happening within your body, not the thoughts popping into your mind. By connecting to your breath, you accomplish two things. First, through inhaling and exhaling deeply, you calm your nervous system. This helps you release any protective emotions such as urgency or resistance and be present with the underlying feeling. Second, connecting with your breath is a way to sink into wherever that emotion is manifesting in your body.

For instance, when I feel anxious, it's like a fluttering sensation that begins in my chest. When I notice something happening in my body, I try to take a breath in and then exhale into where I'm sensing the anxiousness. This allows me to observe more characteristics of what anxiousness is like when it's happening inside me. I might see that it rises with pressure up through my throat, and I will use my breathing to relax into that part of the anxiousness. When I witness anxiousness, or any other emotion, I notice that it's just a series of harmless sensations in a particular part of my body. Contrary to what my brain tells me about anxiousness, nothing terrible will come of allowing it to be inside my body. I won't die from feeling anxious.

Staying focused on what's happening within your body, where the feeling is happening, helps you detach from your mind. The reason feelings such as anxiousness, boredom, or disappointment feel so terrible is only because you're in your head instead of your body. By default, when we first start trying to make sense of our emotions, we tend to rationalize what's happening instead of connecting to the physical sensation itself. Or, instead of noticing what the sensation of the emotion is actually like in the body, we spend time asking ourselves why we feel this way.

This is a common misstep in the early stages of developing emotional awareness. Spending time thinking about the reasons you feel the way you do only works to exacerbate the emotion instead of allowing it to work its way through and out of your body.

The same is true with the physical sensation of hunger. By itself, hunger might feel like some tension below your rib cage, or a cramping movement lower in your belly. Maybe you observe some growling that comes and goes. Just paying attention to these basic sensations is quite manageable by itself.

But when you start thinking you're ravenous, or that something awful will happen if you don't eat in the next five minutes, the hunger intensifies. You intensify the experience of hunger by thinking it's a problem that needs to be solved immediately. Instead, when you observe yourself thinking more about the sensation instead of just describing its physical characteristics, gently remind yourself to drop back into your body.

This is a type of active meditation that brings awareness to the natural language of your body. The more you intentionally practice observing your feelings with detachment from your thoughts, the easier it is to identify your emotions as they crop up during the day. This gives you the chance to pause before reacting from the emotion.

For instance, many of us innately believe that feeling hungry is a problem—a signal from the body that needs to be answered immediately. We've been taught that we should snack throughout the day so we never allow ourselves to get hungry. We want to avoid getting hungry so we don't lower our metabolism. Thoughts like these lead us to think that hunger is an emergency when it's not.

Even after years of doing this work, I occasionally fall into the same trap when I feel hungry. For example, recently we planned to order takeout for dinner. My husband was in charge of ordering and picking up the food since I have a busy schedule with client calls. Now, I like to eat early, and usually I'm in charge of making dinner so it's ready around 5:00 pm. Well, when I ended my last call at 5:00 p.m., I noticed that my husband was hanging out with one of our kids, and the food order hadn't been placed yet.

I knew I was physically hungry, but I also started to feel restless on top of that. I could feel my thoughts racing, believing I couldn't wait another hour to eat, and internally chastising my husband for not picking up the food yet. In my body, I felt the growling of hunger, but I also sensed a fast, antsy energy that I know to be urgency.

Once I sensed that urge, which is the emotion of desire, I was able to bring my awareness back to what was happening in my body. I took a long breath and worked to relax myself with every exhale. I reminded myself that everything was fine, and when I was able to release the urgency, I drew my focus back to hunger itself. When I'm present just with hunger, I'm reminded that the sensations in my stomach are mild and something I can be with for another hour if I need to.

Now, the point isn't to keep delaying hunger. It's to let go of the sense of urgency that often comes along with it based on your thinking. You'll notice that when you delay hunger too long without eating, other physical symptoms begin. You might feel light-headed, distracted, or low on physical energy. These symptoms are much different from the restless feeling of urgency. When you notice the symptoms of prolonged hunger and realize you need to prioritize eating, it's a practical instead of an emotional response to hunger. The energy is very different.

Getting good at separating urgency from true hunger is an important skill to master. It goes a long way to change the tendency of overeating, and it helps you develop more of a comfortable relationship with hunger.

Hunger and satiety are also part of the natural language of your body that you need to learn to interpret and respond to with love. You know now that hunger is not actually a problem or sign that something is wrong. It's just your body having a dialogue with you about what it needs. Your body is not demanding you feed it; it's just letting you know it could use some kind of sustenance.

If food is not the sustenance you give it, your body also knows what to do next to provide you with energy. It will tap into its fat stores. It will utilize your reserves through stored fat on your body, and it will burn them as fuel. Your body is designed to do that, so know that if you choose to sit with hunger instead of eating right away, nothing will go wrong.

Developing a harmonious relationship with hunger is also really helpful in better understanding satiety. Not eating unless you're hungry not only makes eating more pleasurable and satisfying, but it also allows you to more easily identify your satiety level. If you're not hungry when you eat, how will you ever know when you're just satisfied with what you've eaten?

Learning the language of satiety is often much more nuanced than understanding hunger. When you begin eating with some hunger in your belly, pay attention to when the hunger begins to fade as you chew your food. In my experience, it doesn't take many bites before I notice the hunger disappear. As hunger exits, satiety comes in. When you pay attention to satiety for the first time, it's often surprising how little food it takes for hunger to dissipate.

Since satiety enters your body like a whisper, it's especially important to do the work of releasing urgency from hunger. Urgency can happen unconsciously, and it adds a quickening to natural hunger. It stems from believing that your hunger is bigger or more intense than normal, along with the false assumption you need to eat more because of it. Hunger doesn't grow or change much when you get back to the base feeling of it without the urgency. Allowing hunger in your body for two hours instead of thirty minutes doesn't change your satiety point.

Yet when you believe you need more food to satisfy the hunger and have urgency on top of natural hunger in your body, you'll notice yourself rushing and eating quickly. This easily leads to eating beyond your natural satiety because you don't give your body the chance to catch up with the speed of your eating. Your digestive system works slowly to absorb the food; it's not at the same rate as quickly spooning food into your mouth.

It's worth noting that you don't need to delay hunger as a tactic for weight loss, so don't misunderstand allowing some hunger in your body with a diet tactic of under-eating and constantly feeling underfed. Hunger is a key part of your body's natural language, and you and your body are on the same team. Hunger is an ally, notifying you when you need nourishment, but it's not demanding anything from you. Hunger is not an emergency that needs to be answered immediately, either. It will have a dialogue with you throughout the day, and when you befriend it, it's much easier to respond without urgency.

Since hunger is an ally in your effort to live your best life and feel incredible in your body, you also don't want to ignore it. When you push off hunger for too long, your body will send some new signals. Often people describe feeling a lack of focus, fatigue, and light-headedness. These signs are very different from urgency. Recognizing the symptoms of prolonged hunger and intentionally eating in response can also be done without urgency.

Making friends with hunger gives you the chance to decide what you feel comfortable with in your body before eating. Beginning a meal with some hunger is really useful, no matter the degree of hunger you decide you want. The first reason is that it heightens the pleasure in eating when you feel physically satisfied. The second reason is that it makes it easier to detect satiety when you begin your meal hungry.

Just like hunger, you can decide what level of satisfaction you want to feel after eating. This may be different depending on the meal and the time of day. It can also change, too. The satiety level I prefer on a typical weekday is different from the satiety I want if it's Thanksgiving. The way I like to think about my ideal satisfaction is finding the perfect balance between optimal pleasure from food and optimal pleasure in my body.

Having a conscious eating experience is fundamental to achieve this. You need to separate the brain chatter from your body's subtle language to distinguish when the delight in food fades and pleasure in your body begins to wane. It's a process of trial and error to observe how your body feels an hour after completing a meal.

When I experimented with my ideal satiety point, I considered how I wanted my body to feel at the end of a meal. Then, when I sat down to eat, I connected to the feeling of hunger in my belly before I took my first bite. As I ate slowly, I observed what happened with my hunger. After several bites, I noticed that hunger faded. Simultaneously, satiety gently made its presence known. At that point, I started asking questions. "How does my body feel? Is this enough?"

You get to decide what level of satisfaction you want to feel. Just know that many people who have a love language of food associate "fullness" with being satisfied. Perhaps you've believed that you're not yet satisfied if you don't feel the weight of fullness in your belly. For the purpose of feeling the best you can in your body, you can determine whether keeping that assumption is helping you.

I know that when clients come to me for help with weight loss, needing to be full is a barrier to getting to their ideal size. To reestablish a new comfort level of satiety, I always recommend that you experiment and stop eating sooner. Sometimes the ideal point for weight loss is just when hunger fades and you begin to question if you're satisfied enough. It's often before you think you've eaten enough.

Listening to the subtle response of your body requires deliberate detachment from your love language with food. Your love language with food will tell you, "Finish every last bite," "You don't want to waste even one delicious piece of this," or "This is all for you." None of those thoughts are connected to what your body needs. They're driven by desire, not pure hunger.

Food for Thought

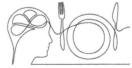

1. Establishing the ideal level of satiety to feel incredible in your body also depends on what you notice after eating. Listen to what's happening in your body an hour after completing a meal and decide how your body feels. Take

note of the heaviness or lightness you experience and the level of energy you have.

2. If it's after your final meal of the day, how does your body feel when you go to sleep? Consider how your sleep itself is affected by the satisfaction in your body.

3. Being attuned to your preferred hunger and satiety levels takes the focus off food and back to where you have all your control. Your body knows what it needs to be feeling its best, and it's waiting for you to listen. What are you hearing your body say to you?

Chapter 13:

The Joy of Missing Out

Food used to be an escape for Synthia. As we worked together, I helped her stop eating for relief during online work meetings. She learned skills to manage urges while getting through stressful project deadlines. In the absence of overeating, Synthia realized that she had overcommitted herself to work and that underneath all her cravings for food was a desperate need for downtime.

The process of changing her relationship with food took time and involved lots of setbacks. But after four months, Synthia not only lost twenty pounds, but also created a more enjoyable life for herself.

Our last meeting was shortly after Synthia returned from a weeklong work conference. Historically, this kind of trip triggered Synthia's old way of relating to food. In the past, she loathed traveling for work since it always led to overindulging in the buffet of snacks at meetings, splurging on dinner when she and her colleagues dined out, and raiding the mini bar in her hotel room before bed.

During my final call with Synthia, I was eager to check in and see how her business trip had gone. It had been a month since our last meeting, and this final call was a chance for the two of us to check her progress. Over our twelve sessions together, she gradually worked to shift her habits toward being more intentional around food. She regularly planned her meals in advance, but she also thought strategically about special events and how to navigate obstacles around them. By this point, she knew enough about her old triggers and the thoughts that usually motivated her to overeat that she could anticipate what her brain would suggest before it even happened.

Within moments of connecting online, I could sense Synthia's delight. Her smile beamed across the screen, and her skin glowed with a radiance I had not seen before in her. Before I could ask her the questions I jotted down before our call, she eagerly started filling me in on the juicy tidbits of her eating over the last few weeks.

"I really enjoyed the conference," she said affirmatively. "Instead of feeling drained, I came home refreshed. It was really a welcome break from my usual routine."

I listened attentively, excited by such a significant shift in her perspective. Synthia used to dread work trips, and the sense of defeat that came from returning home physically and mentally weighed her down. Every time she traveled for work, she gained several pounds, and she routinely avoided the scale for several weeks after the trip ended. The pattern of mindless eating on work trips and the cycle of guilt and defeat on the back end led to constant frustration and hopelessness. But during this last conversation with Synthia, her usual disappointment in herself was replaced with excitement. She was cheerful and effervescent as she shared the details with me.

"What was different this time?" I asked.

"I just focused a lot less on the food," she replied. "I decided I would enjoy the people and the experience more than eating, and it felt really freeing."

That freedom is what I heard in Synthia's voice. There was a levity in her disposition, and her eyes sparkled with life.

Synthia recounted how she didn't restrict herself with food but instead made the intentional choice to only indulge in foods she would thoroughly enjoy. Because she wasn't trying to be strict with herself, she felt more empowered to make thoughtful choices. The conference was at a fancy resort with delicious eating options, and Synthia opted to have small amounts of some of her favorite foods. By not trying to lose weight, follow her plan perfectly, or be too strict with herself, she took the pressure off and felt more empowered.

"I realized after my first day of the conference that I could really do this," she said to me confidently. "I had just enough of some of my favorite foods, but I also loved how much better my body felt not overeating."

Synthia's confidence gave her momentum throughout the trip to act in alignment with her commitment to herself. Instead of feeling obligated to eat out with a large group every night, she stayed in a couple of nights and enjoyed a quiet evening to herself. Without feeling weighed down mentally and physically by extra eating, Synthia had the energy to wake up early and hit the gym in the hotel.

"I can't remember the last time I felt like exercising on a work trip," she admitted on our call. "But fitting into some of my favorite outfits, and knowing I was in control of how much I ate, made the trip a lot more fun."

What's more, Synthia maintained her weight instead of gaining a few pounds. It was easy to transition back to her core way of eating because she felt so inspired by her progress.

Synthia's example is proof that there can be joy in missing out on extra eating. When she took the emphasis off food as the source of her pleasure, she discovered ways to have fun, relax, connect, and be energized that promoted a longer-lasting sense of well-being. Her success at the work conference was the direct result of her willingness to unlearn old habits and practice new ones over the course of several months working with me. The journey began by changing her normal routine at home and noticing patterns of escaping with food.

Week by week, she paid attention to her body and realized how much more alive she felt when she properly nourished herself. She built trust in her ability to make decisions around food and follow through on them. She slowly learned which foods she enjoyed and felt good in her body. She did the emotional work of honoring her feelings and making space for them instead of distracting herself with food, and her mood improved. She felt more and more capable of navigating difficult experiences and knowing how to support herself through them. As her body responded with more energy, lightness, and a newfound vibrancy, Synthia discovered the joy of reconnecting with her authentic self.

The joy Synthia discovered in herself was a deeply satisfying one. The fleeting pleasure of a bite of chocolate or glass of wine is nothing compared to the experience of thoroughly quenching the thirst of your soul. For the first time in her life, Synthia was able to answer the question "What am I still hungry for?" and fully satisfy it. Once she tasted the joy of missing out, there was no forgetting the soothing peace that washed over her mind, body, and spirit. She replaced her desire for more food with a yearning to continue loving herself.

Like most of my clients, it took Synthia time to change the habit of overeating. It was a process of practicing, failing, learning from setbacks, and then recommitting to herself. Without the distraction of work or food to fill the void, she became more acquainted with her feelings and her core needs. She rediscovered her authentic self and learned how to respond differently to her desire.

Synthia used to think that work was the problem and traveling was the cause of her weight gain. But ultimately she learned there was more she wanted from her life—and her daily routine needed to change to honor that. When we explored what made the work trips so difficult, a big reason was that Synthia didn't enjoy herself. She felt weighed down by all the extra eating and usually returned home stressed out by the experience. When food was such a big distraction from herself, she didn't have the physical or mental energy to be as productive in her job or thoroughly enjoy herself outside of work.

Figuring out how to master work trips without eating too much was a huge win for Synthia. "I never felt overly full or deprived," she told me. "It was the best of both worlds, because

I enjoyed the flavor of food while still feeling good in my body." As a result, Synthia felt confident in her ability to honor herself and stayed committed to eating mindfully for the entire week of the trip. She described the excitement she experienced wearing some of her favorite outfits—outfits that previously didn't fit when she was overeating. She felt connected to her colleagues, had energy to exercise in the mornings, and slept peacefully in the hotel every evening. "It felt like a mini vacation," Synthia said. Instead of needing to recover from the conference, she returned home revitalized, with a renewed sense of commitment to herself.

How would you describe the pleasure of eating less? How does life become more joyful when some of the food you're currently eating is off the table?

I like to pose these two questions to people who tell me they just love food so much and have a hard time stopping at less. I hear from my clients that the mental chatter around food, daydreaming about food, and the frustration with themselves over eating too much is all-consuming. They've had enough of it, and they want to be done with all the energy, time, and focus this relationship costs them. But they don't know how to change. They feel powerless around the pull to nibble, snack, or go in for one more bite.

When you have a big emotional appetite, you're used to believing that you're missing out if you're not able to enjoy *all* the food.

By this point in the book, you've probably figured out the role of your emotional appetite and how all the attractive thoughts you have about food have led to an abundant desire for it. It may seem like if you're not eating, there is less pleasure, joy, and fun in life.

But what if that's not true?

The more you think that food is what you want to feel better and enjoy yourself more, naturally you'll desire more food. But if you're reading this book, and you're dissatisfied with life, your body, or how the way you eat makes you feel, you want to pay attention here. As much as your brain tells you in the moment that you want food, your current results are showing you that you don't—at least not the same amount of food.

If your current way of eating is creating discomfort and a lower quality of life, food isn't making you feel better; it's making you feel worse.

Your brain is not always a truth teller, in case you haven't noticed. It's driven to perpetuate old habits that create instant gratification, even when those old habits are at the expense of your long-term health.

Your brain is confused about food. It will lead you to believe that more is better, because with every dopamine rush it gets from a piece of cake or sip of wine, it thinks that pleasure must indicate you need those things to survive. Your brain will lead you to believe that it's a good idea to escape feelings of boredom with food, so you never teach yourself how to manage and soothe your emotions. Emotions, when you're inexperienced at feeling them, seem like unfamiliar territory to your brain. That unfamiliar territory is interpreted as scary and dangerous for survival. Your primal brain doesn't understand that learning to listen to your emotions will make you more secure instead of less.

When food is your love language, you spend quite a lot of time building up your desire to eat, so the idea of eating less probably seems less compelling.

But to create a relationship with food and your body that harmoniously maximizes the pleasure in both, you need to start creating the desire for less food.

So where do you start? The answer may not seem obvious right now.

You start with where you are and telling yourself the full truth about your current relationship with food.

If giving into every impulse to eat leads you to feel bloated, lethargic, and weighed down, remind yourself of that. If certain foods give you indigestion, make you feel restless, or don't really satisfy your hunger, make yourself aware of that. You need to begin with reminding yourself of the truth that over-eating does not truly make things better for you in the long run. Telling yourself the honest truth will help to lessen your desire for all the food.

The next step is to experiment with having foods you know feel good in your body and eating them according to your body's natural language. Don't think of this as a weight-loss tactic. It's more of an opportunity to be in harmony with your body without ending your love of food. It's a chance to honor both while prioritizing your own well-being above all else. Taking the emphasis off weight loss helps keep the focus on your body and how you want to be feeling. That's where the focus needs to be if you want to experience the joy of missing out.

Start to notice the change in how you feel when you practice honoring the internal language of your body, instead of pursuing your love language of food. Let's say you stop eating something delicious as soon as you notice you're no longer physically hungry—at the very beginning of satiety and before you feel fullness. What do you notice about your body?

It probably feels lighter and more energized. Instead of needing to take a nap, you might be able to get things done during your day or simply enjoy the calmness in your digestion. When you take a break from eating all the food, you start to experience a new kind of pleasure. It's the pleasure of feeling better you always thought you'd get from the extra food. But now you begin to see how feeling better comes less from pursuing food and more from honoring your body.

It is a joyful experience to feel effervescent in your body when you're charged with energy, feel light instead of weighed down with food, and have the mental clarity of not obsessing about food. There is a deep level of pleasure in sitting down for a meal of your favorite indulgent foods, having a nice glass of wine, easily leaving some of the food and wine behind on your plate because you are fully satisfied with less, and confident in stopping without clearing your plate. Imagine the joy in using the extra energy and focus you used to devote to eating to pursuing a lifelong dream. Maybe it's creating a piece of art, building a business, completing an endurance race, or learning a new skill.

When you engage in the love language of food, you might assume you're missing out if you can't have all the available food. But food is not going anywhere, my friend. In case you haven't noticed, it's abundant. There are delicious things to eat around every corner. If you really want to indulge in something tasty, the opportunities are not running out, contrary to what your brain is telling you.

But there is a finite amount of time to create the life you want for yourself. Chasing the next delicious bite only leads to more of the same—a life devoted to food. The love language of food leads to a lifestyle of consumption rather than creation, and that consumption never feels deeply gratifying, in a soulful kind of way.

Recognizing the joy and pleasure that comes from eating the ideal way for your body is a necessary aspect of maintaining this new relationship with food. The more you appreciate the pleasure in how light and energized your body feels, the more likely you are to desire that. I began with noticing how certain foods felt in my body when I ate them according to my natural signals of hunger and satiety. I observed how some meats created a heaviness, while others didn't. Some types of beans created a gurgling effect in my stomach I didn't like, while lentils helped me feel grounded and cozy. I worked to cultivate more of a feeling of being grounded in my body by eating foods that settled well and created easy digestion.

It was easy to eat in a way that was pleasurable and also satisfying when I focused on making my body feel well. This naturally lessened my desire for things that upset that happy balance. It's not that I stopped eating certain foods just for fun, but I definitely want them a lot less than before. When I eat certain foods just for fun instead of for any nutritional value, I'm really intent on getting the full flavor from the experience of eating them, but without upsetting the pleasure in my body.

Cooking is a delightful experience when you no longer need to eat or drink your way through the experience. Perhaps in the past, you've believed having a glass of wine or grazing on all the ingredients while preparing a meal genuinely made it more enjoyable. But these things only distract from your ability to be fully present to the joy of creating a meal that's nourishing to the mind, body, and spirit. Engaging in the texture of vegetables as I chop them, the sound of meat sizzling in a pan, or the aroma of soup wafting from its pot is a cheery experience. I can feel satisfied and relaxed after thirty minutes of cooking without taking one bite of the surrounding food. When I'm ready to sit down and enjoy the fruits of my labor, I enjoy the pleasure more of eating what I've cooked from a place of real hunger.

Some of the joy in missing out on all the food is knowing you no longer need more food to be satisfied. The new kind of satisfaction you have comes from feeling amazing in your body. To not struggle with wearing clothes you love, to have the mobility to use your body the way you want to, and to be content with less of your favorite food are all so much more rewarding for most people than having another bite. Disrobing the guilt and shame that comes from feeling powerless around food creates the space to be outwardly joyful and enjoy your relationship with yourself more.

When you purposefully "miss out" on or opt out of having food beyond your ideal satiety level, there is no sense of deprivation; instead, there is a deep-seated peace. When you experience JOMO, it's after you've built up your desire to feel incredible in your body, so much so that the pull toward food has all but disappeared. There isn't the wanting from a large emotional appetite to eat more because the idea of feeling uncomfortable in your body is so unappetizing. When my clients go through this transformation from believing a slice of chocolate cake is their absolute favorite food to really not wanting it anymore, it feels miraculous. They might decide to have some on purpose, but they only desire a few bites in order to preserve the sense of pleasure in their body.

Choosing to not eat all the food that's available rewards you with the joy of being at peace within your body and mind. The joy of being integrity with your emotions (instead of eating to avoid them) and body (instead of overriding its natural signals of hunger and satiety) is a feeling of ease and freedom. It's what I often describe as freedom around food. It liberates you from the tyranny of obsessing about food and your body, and it brings you back to a place of harmony with what your body wanted in the first place.

Conclusion:

The Freedom

B y this point in the book, you've probably realized, just like I did, that food is not the problem, and it's not the answer. It's just a convenient distraction that can easily be labeled and blamed until it consumes much more focus and energy than it deserves. For an inanimate object, it's interesting how food can be the source of so much passion and angst in one person's lifetime.

Like many of the clients I've worked with, you might be disappointed to learn that food is not your friend. You may even be saddened to part with it once you discover how little of it you genuinely need to feel your best. On the other side of mourning, the loss of food is an invitation to get to know yourself. Sadness around losing the comfort of food may just be the first opportunity to nurture and support yourself in an emotionally satisfying way.

One of my most favorite clients once told me, "Weight loss is merely a side effect of me learning how to honor and take care of myself." Many of us food lovers realize, after years of over-eating, that more is not always better when it comes to food. Our bodies rebel, our mental health suffers, and happiness eludes us no matter how much we chase down the next delicious lick, bite, or sip. There is no denying the truth of the body when it's ready to be reckoned with.

This is not a one-size-fits-all approach to slimming for the sake of vanity. There is nothing wrong with wanting to look your best, by the way. But when the aftermath of too much eating and drinking wreaks havoc on your well-being, redefining your approach to eating is about so much more than getting to your goal weight. For me, the journey began with the belief that I deserved to feel better. I took the first step toward ending my love affair with food because I owed it to myself, and I believed my family deserved to have the best version of me by their side. The path forward was full of temptations, doubt, disappointment, confusion, and plenty of opportunities to give up. Giving up always felt like such an easy way out.

But my body knew better, and once I tasted the freedom that came with understanding my emotions, trusting myself, and feeling revitalized in my body, the desire to turn back my old friend food switched from a roaring fire into a flickering flame. It drew me back less and less every time. The allure of food and alcohol is still very real, and it's not going anywhere. Each of us lives every day with the attractive feed of tantalizing images popping up on social media, splashed across television, and paraded around storefronts. If we're not careful, we may even believe that food is the answer to more fun, more connection, and a soul-satisfying experience. But food never promised you any of those things, and at the bottom of the bowl, there are no answers—only more questions.

We all have an innate desire to be happy and comfortable. For many of us, food pretends to fill the void until it becomes obvious that it can't. Think of this book as a road map to discovering what truly satisfies you in a deeply soulful way. There is no timeline to this process or set goal that will validate that you've arrived at the finish line. It is simply a practice of showing up for yourself every single day and recommitting to your best self. Be willing to pull up a seat at the table and meet yourself where you are. Explore the full platter of your emotions and feast on musings of your heart. Embrace your body, honor your physical hunger, and redefine what it means to be fed enough.

Acknowledgments

The journey of self-discovery is a lifelong one. In my process of unraveling a love affair with food and wine, I unearthed my authentic self and the emotions buried beneath years of eating for comfort. My story began with a passion for food and connection and continues to be a process of understanding and honoring my deepest needs. Food continues to be a source of pleasure and joy that connects me to others equally as passionate about living their best lives.

This book is first the result of my own willingness to listen and honor my own inner knowing. I know this intuition as the Holy Spirit, who is advocating on my behalf to become more of my authentic self. This truth prompted me to reconsider how I ate and drank several years before I was brave enough to begin the journey. For that I am eternally thankful.

Learning how to reconnect to my physical and emotional needs was the foundation of changing my relationship with food and alcohol. This work could not have been possible without the guidance and mentorship of several key coaches. I am indebted to Kathryn Green, Laura Dixon, and Nicky Hammond for helping me make sense of old habits, dismantle old beliefs, and be empowered through a new mindset.

Once I discovered how to combine a love of food with a process of losing weight, it was a matter of testing it on like-minded food lovers who were eager to feel and look their best. I learned as much from my clients as I did from my own weight-loss journey about the core reasons people turn to food and the common reasons we struggle to honor our bodies. I am so grateful to each and every one of my clients (you know who you are) who were vulnerable and brave enough to share their journey of weight loss with me. It's an honor and privilege I hold very dear.

Without the support of my family, none of this would be possible. First and foremost, thanks to my husband, Alex, who encouraged and supported me through this project from the beginning. Also, to my father, Peter, who was my first coach and always believed I was capable of more. Finally, to my mother, Jan, for never making any food off-limits and encouraging me to pursue my dream of becoming a chef.

To the Morgan James Publishing team: thank you to founder and CEO David Hancock for supporting this project and helping it reach the hands of countless food lovers. Thanks also to my Author Relations Manager, Emily Madison, for streamlining the process and making it easy to publish this book.

And thanks to my editor and advisor Amanda Rooker and her team at Split Seed Media, for their guidance and patience in crafting the manuscript.

About the Author

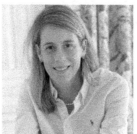

Molly Zemek is a Master Certified Life Coach and professionally trained chef. Her coaching helps food lovers rediscover joy in their bodies without giving up delicious things to eat. She is the host of the podcast *Weight Loss for Food Lovers* and lives in McLean, Virginia, with her husband and three sons. Read more at her website: www.mollyzemek.com.

A free ebook edition is available with the purchase of this book.

To claim your free ebook edition:

1. Visit MorganJamesBOGO.com
2. Sign your name CLEARLY in the space
3. Complete the form and submit a photo of the entire copyright page
4. You or your friend can download the ebook to your preferred device

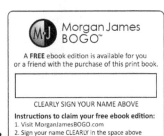

Morgan James
BOGO™

A **FREE** ebook edition is available for you or a friend with the purchase of this print book.

CLEARLY SIGN YOUR NAME ABOVE

Instructions to claim your free ebook edition:
1. Visit MorganJamesBOGO.com
2. Sign your name CLEARLY in the space above
3. Complete the form and submit a photo of this entire page
4. You or your friend can download the ebook to your preferred device

Print & Digital Together Forever.

Snap a photo

Free ebook

Read anywhere

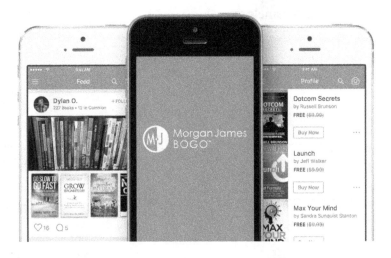

Printed in the USA
CPSIA information can be obtained
at www.ICGtesting.com
JSHW020948250224
57970JS00002B/31